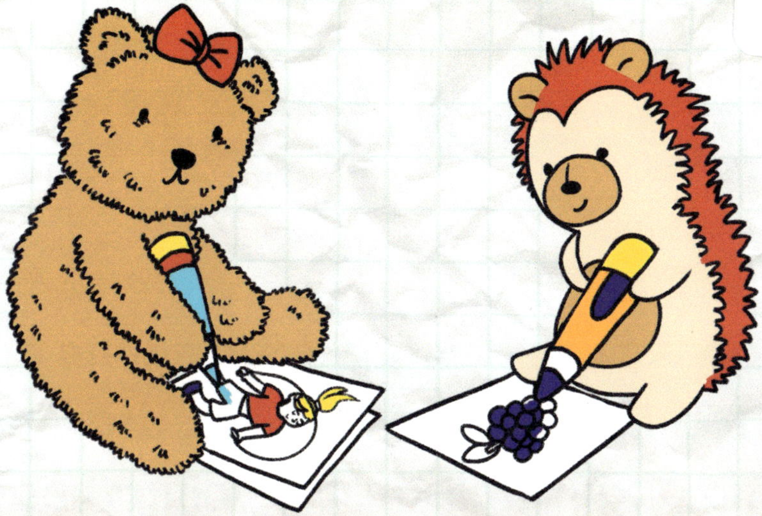

CLUB Member Name:

warmBLUSH

by Kendrick W. Monestime, MHA

From the creators of the
"Somebody Needs This" Well-being Podcast

note to parents

warmBLUSH books are designed for adults and parents to interact with children while reading, drawing, coloring, and learning about well-being. Doing these activities together is a magnificent experience, and an opportunity to teach little ones about taking care of their well-being.

THANK YOU

to all of our parents, kids, and adults who take the time to

REVIEW our books on Amazon.

Reviews really help us to better serve you.

Visit

www.WARMBLUSH.com

From the creators of the
"Somebody Needs This" Well-being Podcast

note to parents

- Fruits and vegetables are classified from both a botanical and culinary standpoint.
- Botanical: Relates to the edible portion of the plant
- Culinary: Relates to how the food is actually consumed
- Therefore, there are vegetables that some people consider fruits, and vice versa.

- In a perfect world, it would be nice to have at least one recognizable fruit and vegetable begin with each letter of the alphabet. However, that is not the case. We would rather people using the book become familiar with fruits and vegetables that can hopefully be accessible to them. So, we do try to mix in some new things. However, at times instead of saying 'F' is for fiddlehead, we'll rather say there is an 'f' in cauliflower.

A

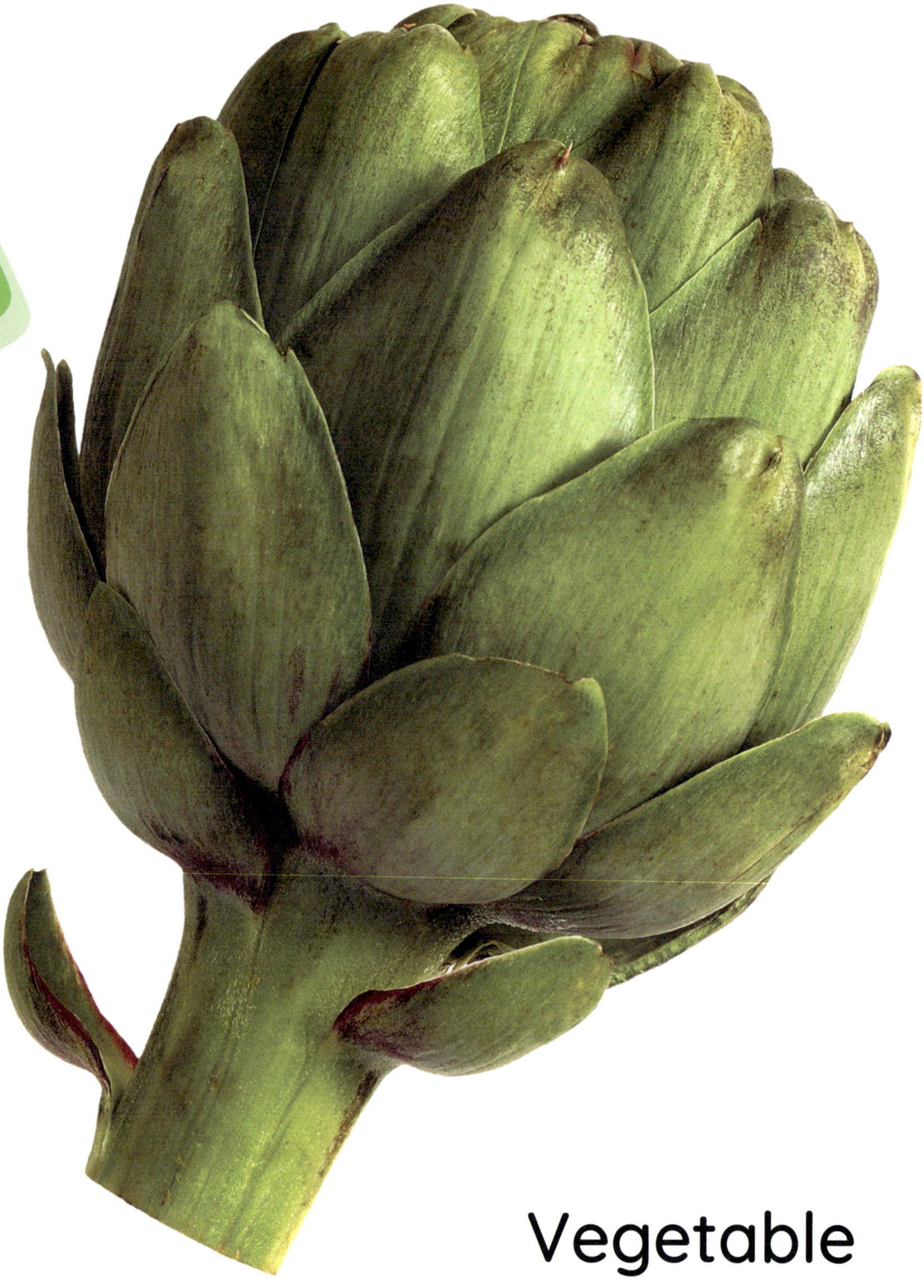

Artichoke

Vegetable

a

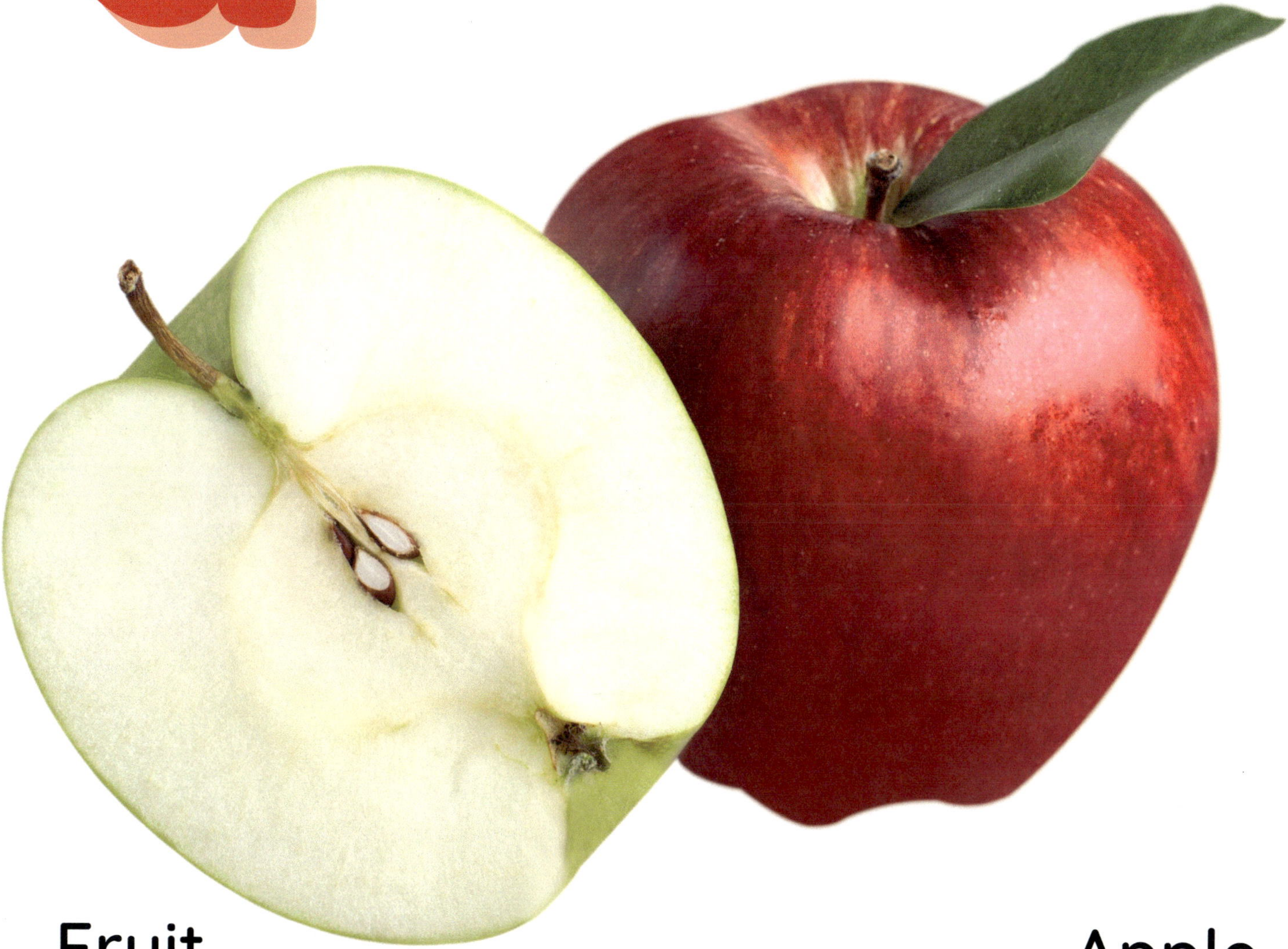

Fruit

Apple

B

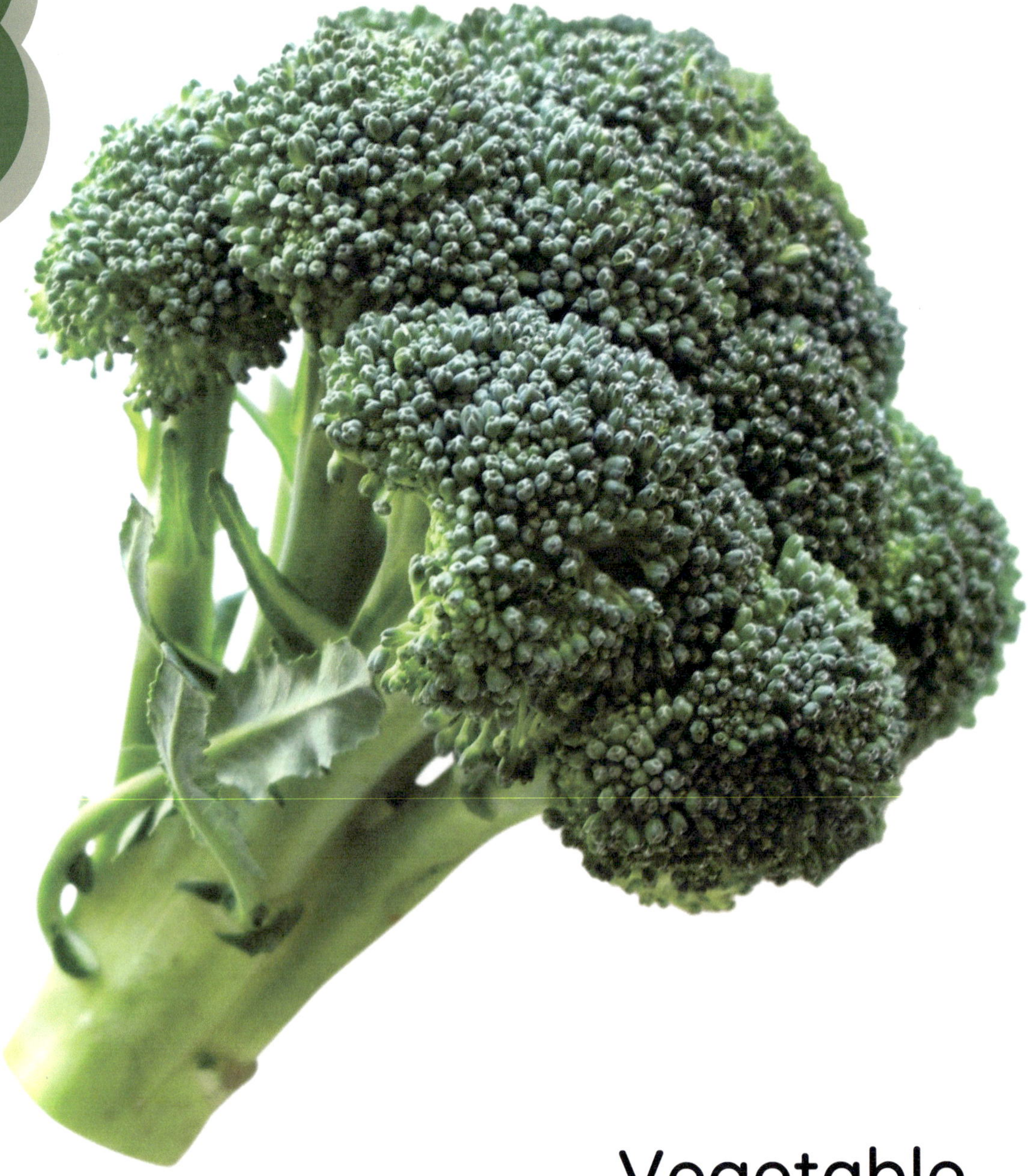

Broccoli

Vegetable

b

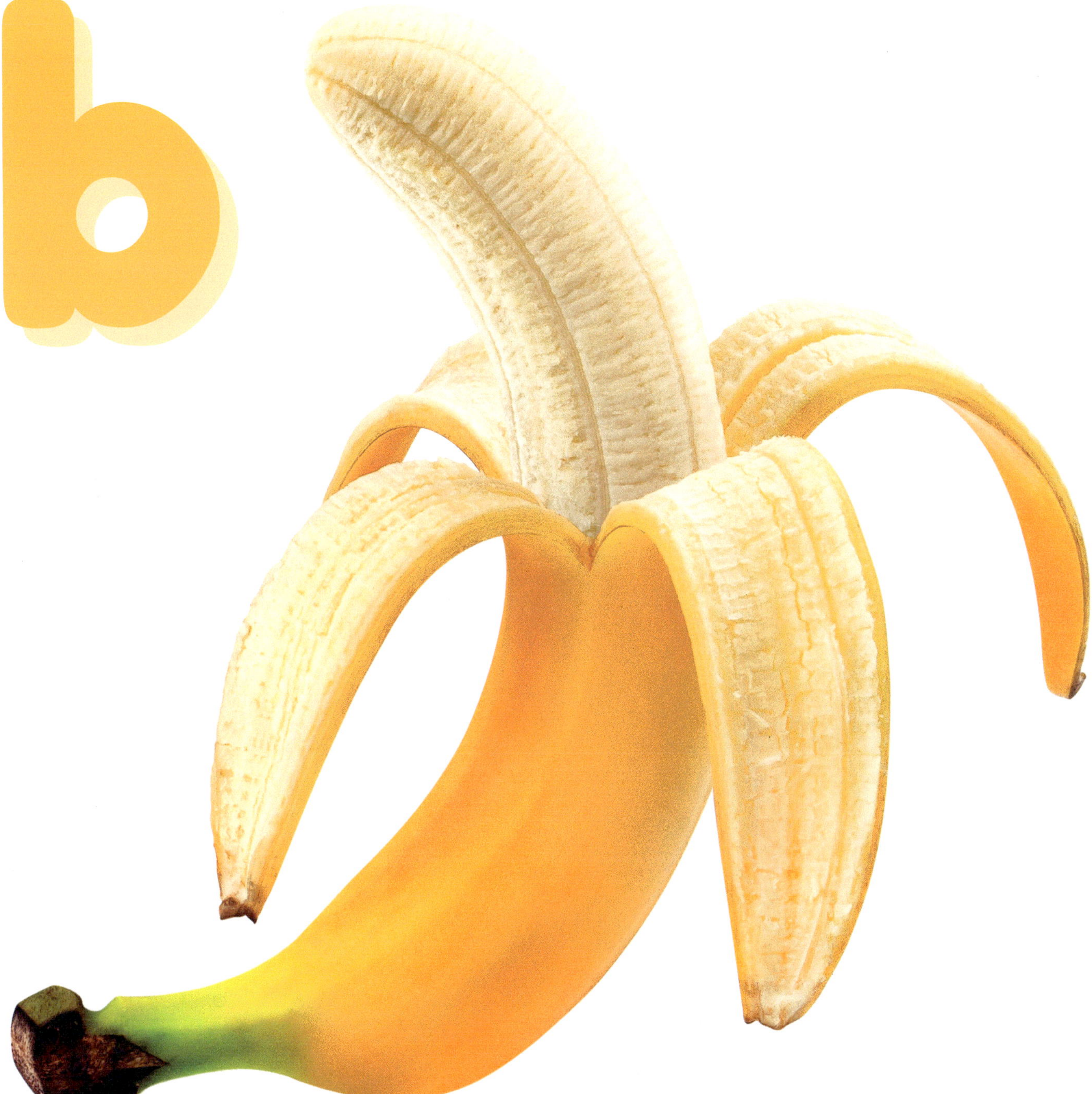

Fruit

Banana

C

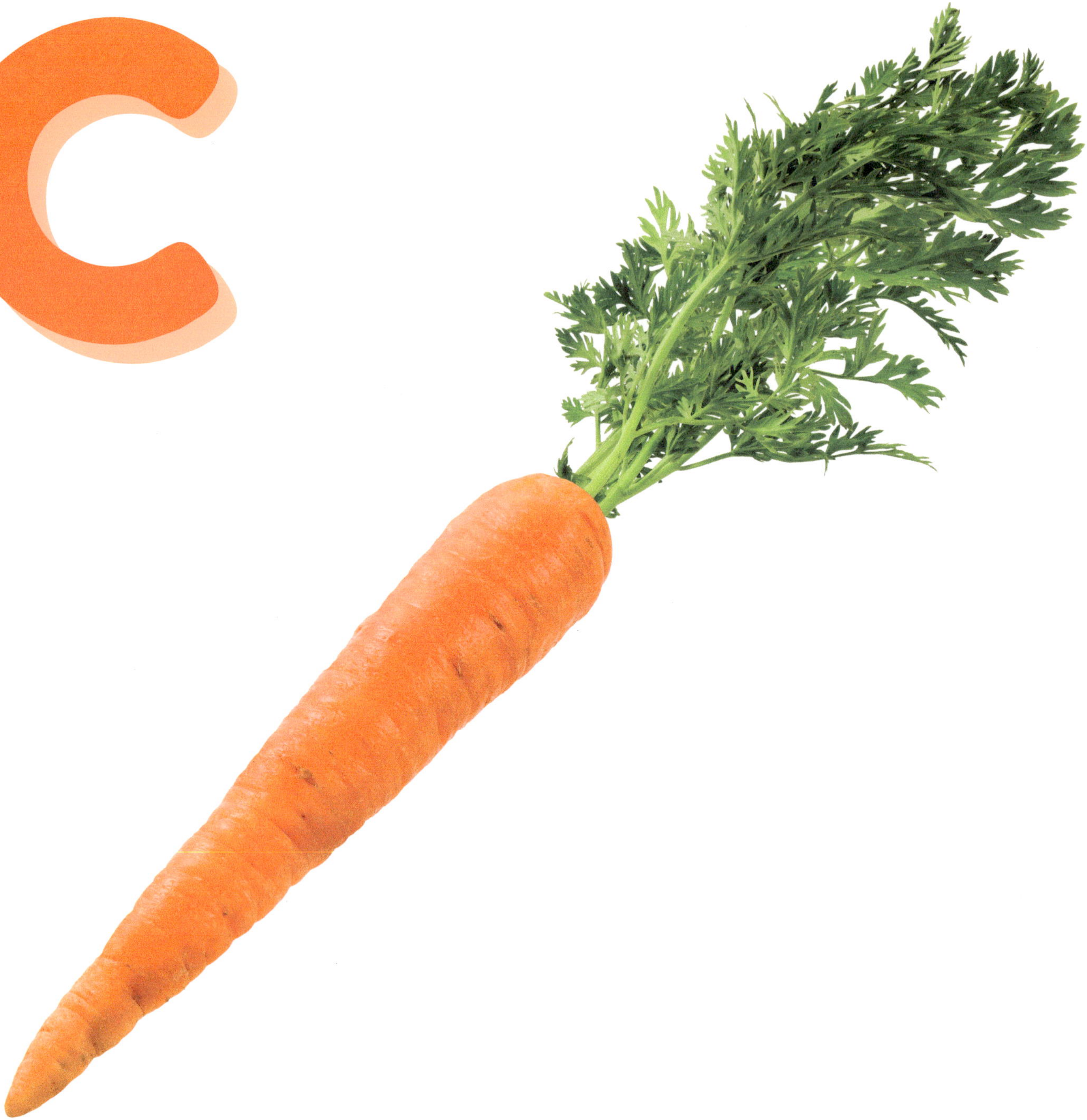

Carrot

Vegetable

C

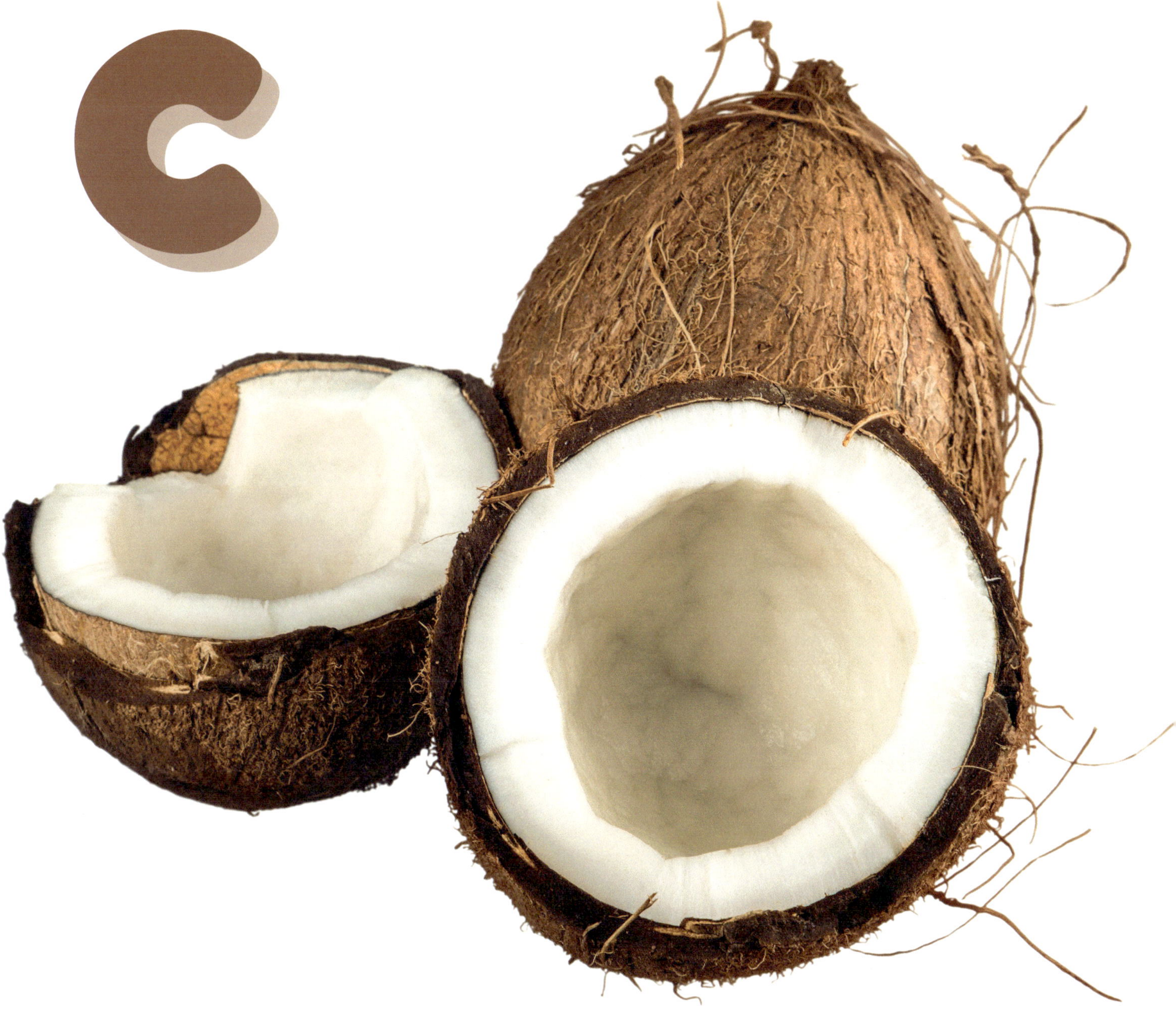

Fruit

Coconut

D

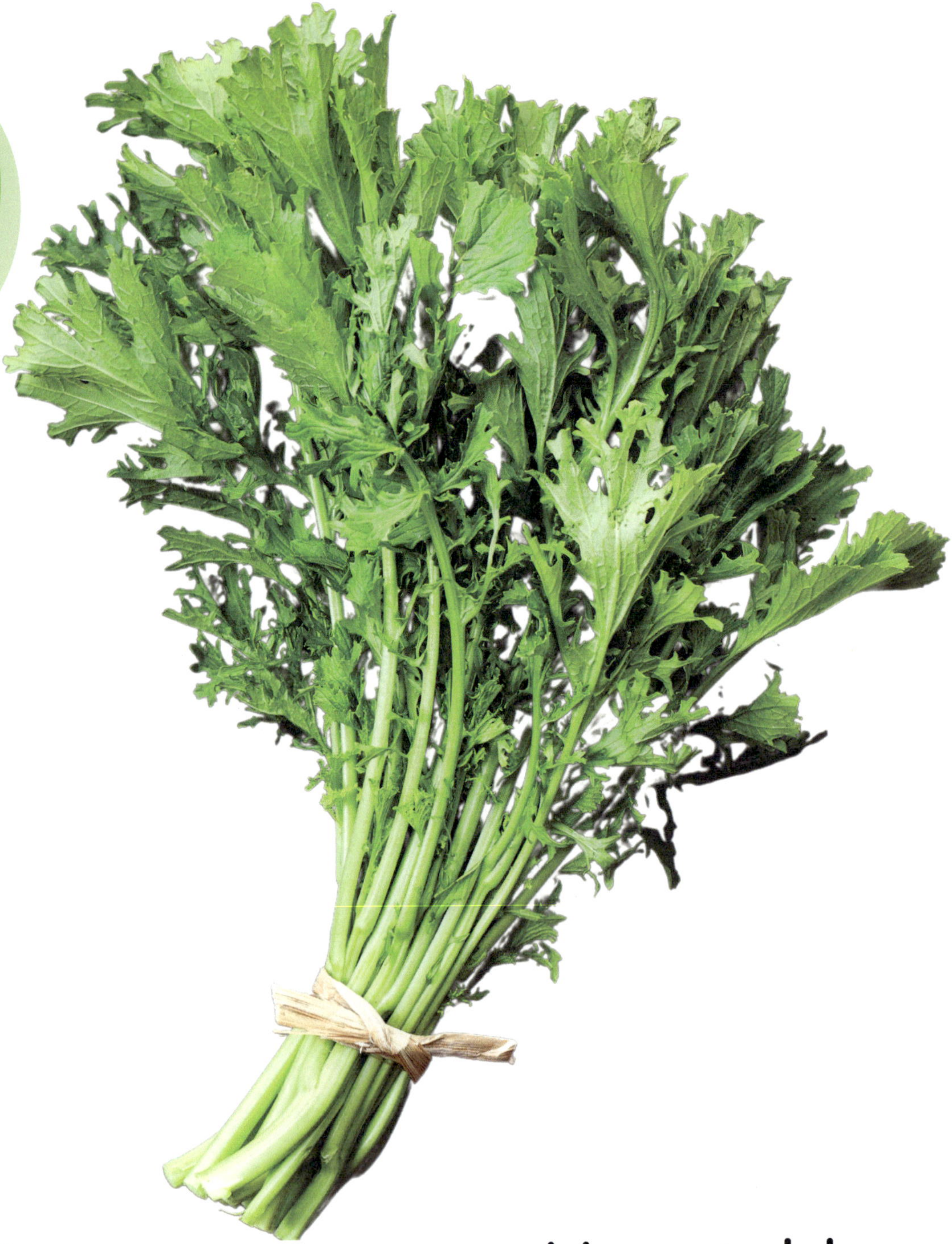

Mustard Greens

Vegetable

d

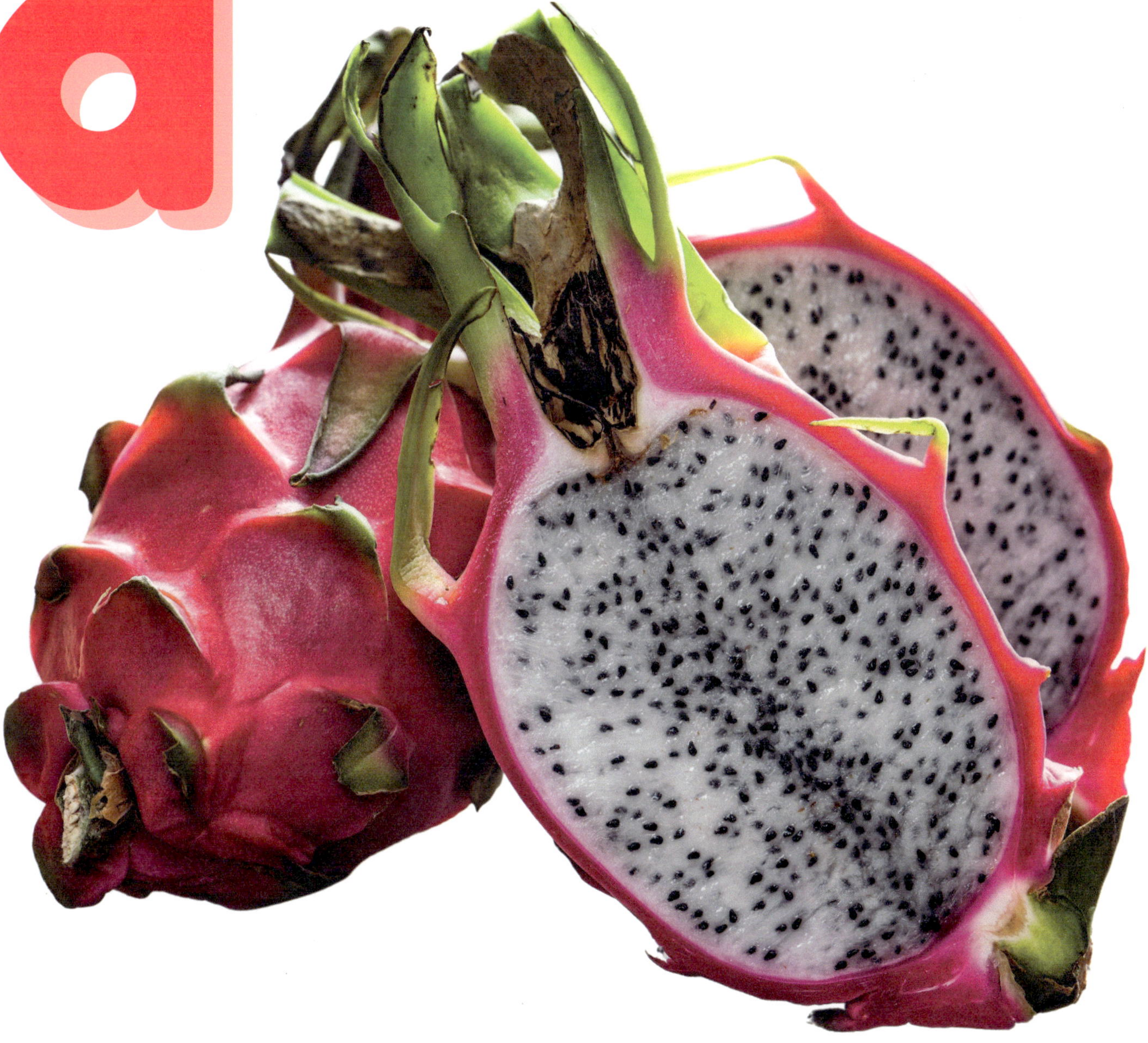

Fruit

Dragonfruit

E

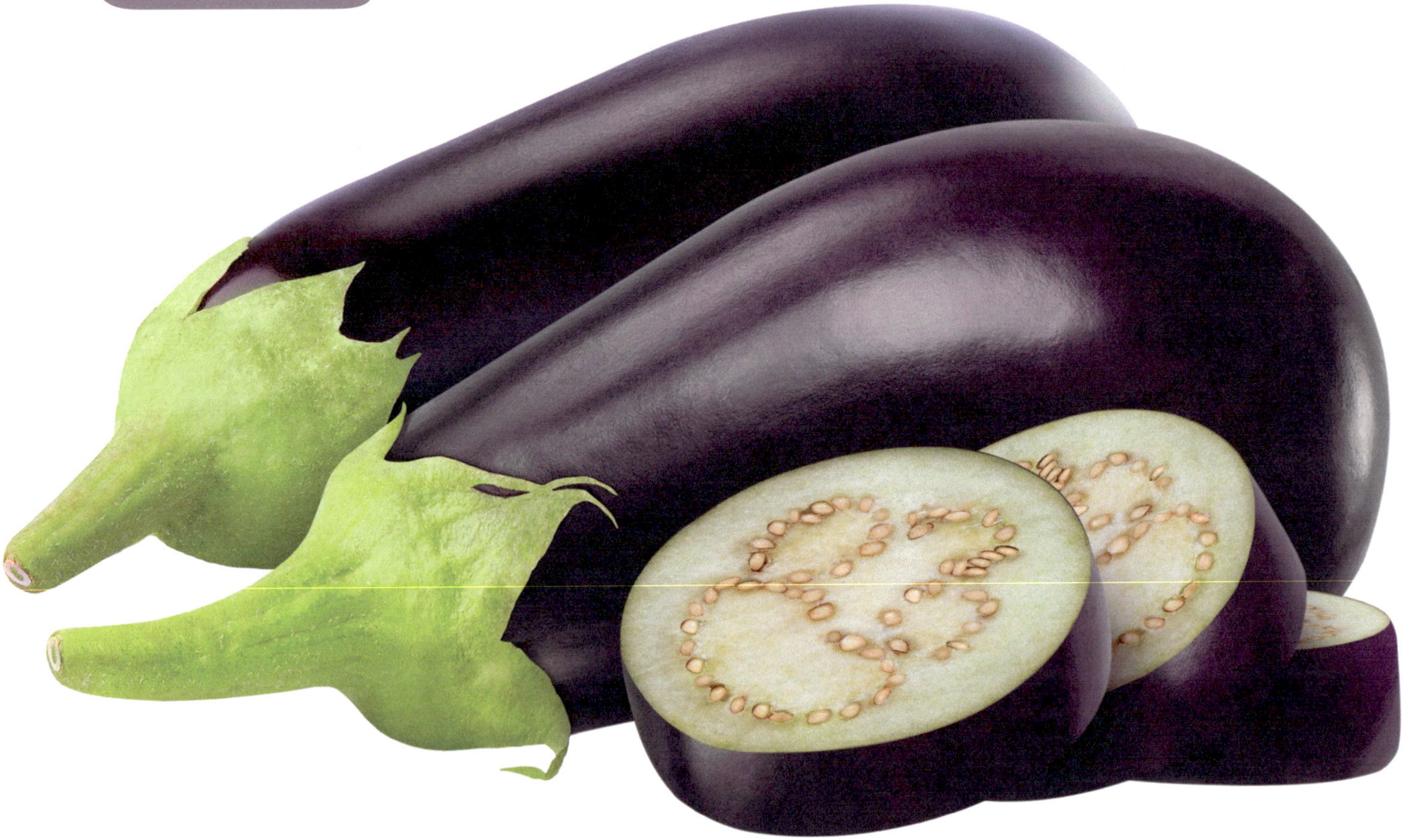

Eggplant

Vegetable

e

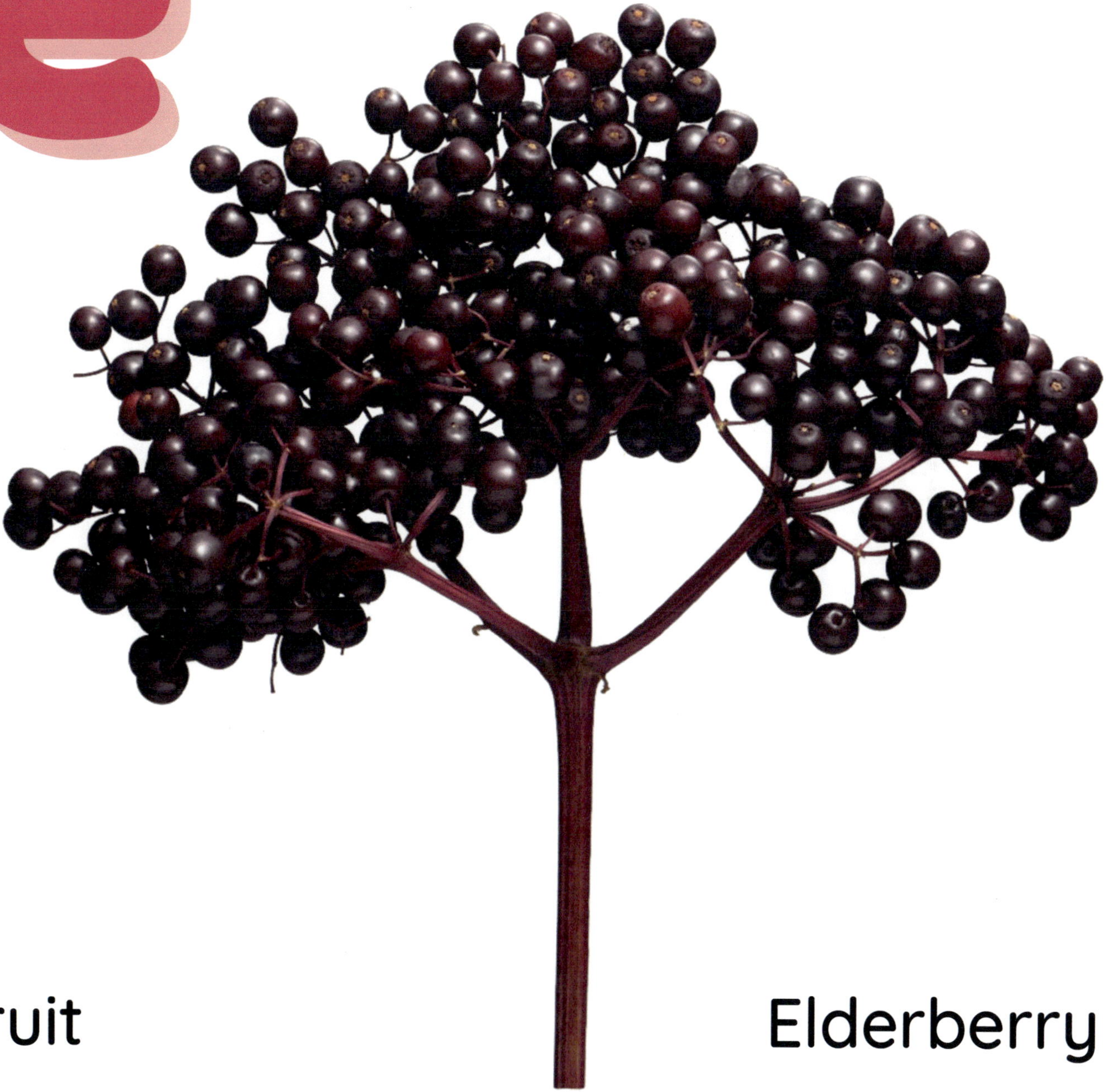

Fruit

Elderberry

F

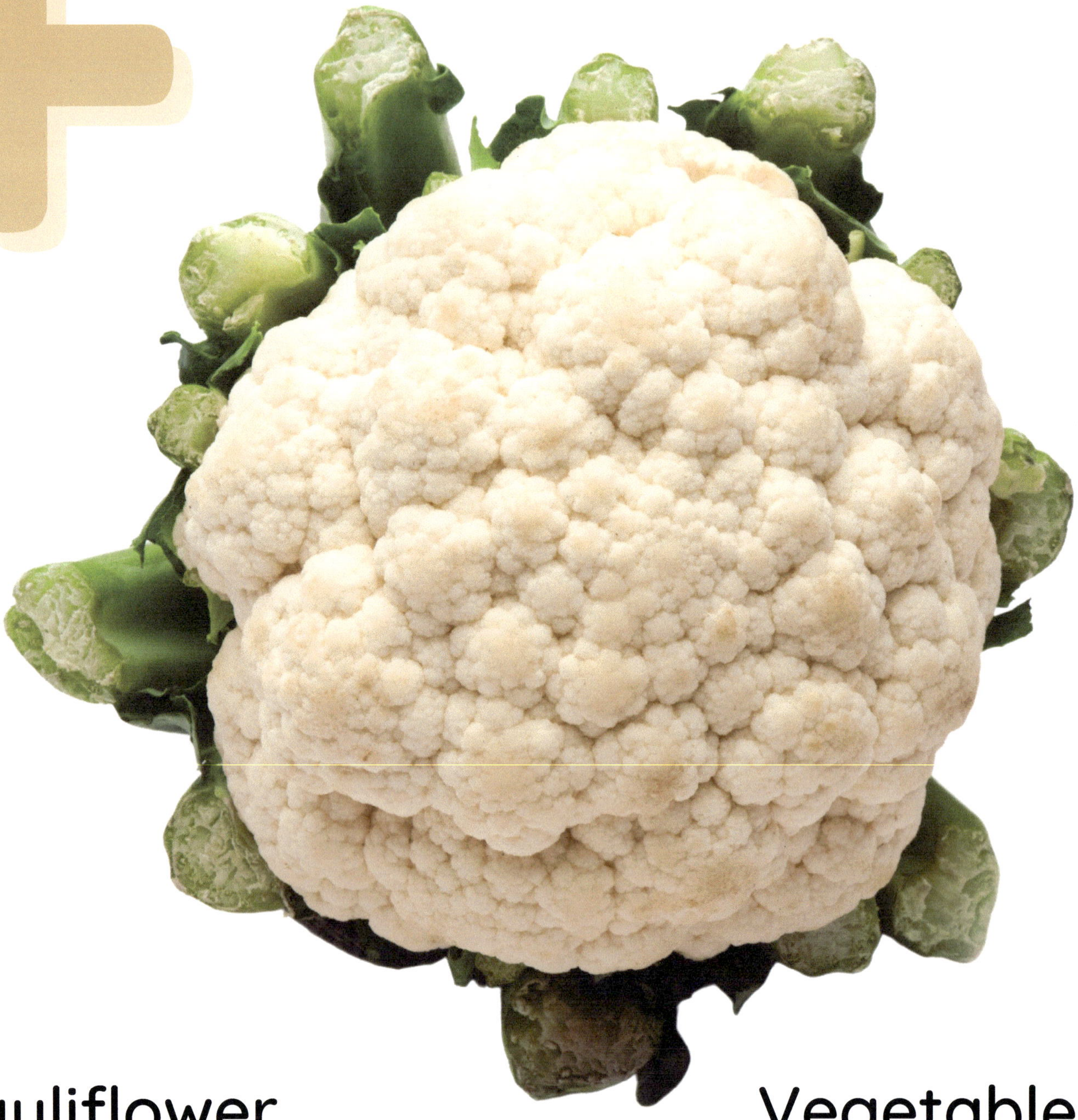

Cauliflower

Vegetable

f

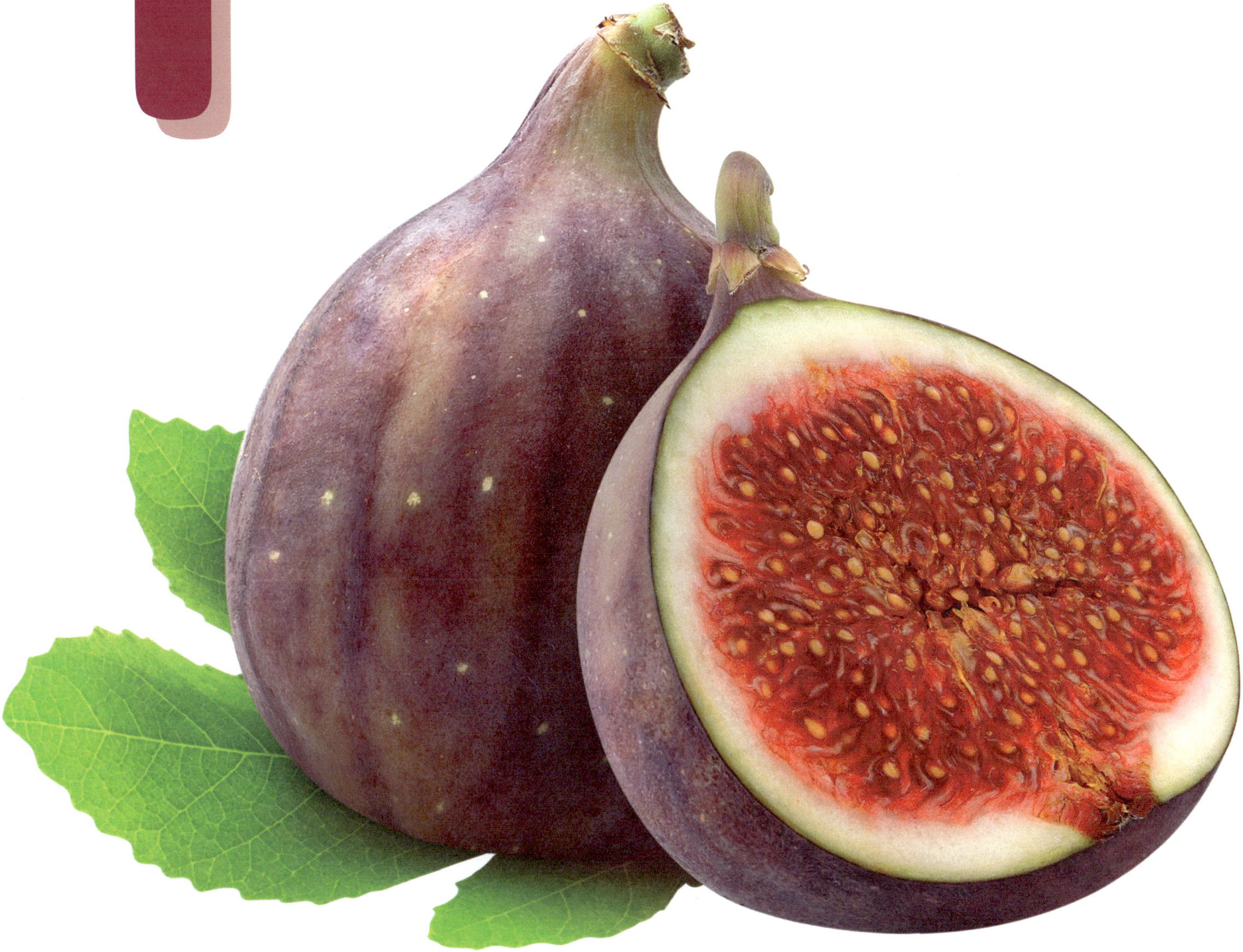

Fruit

Figs

G

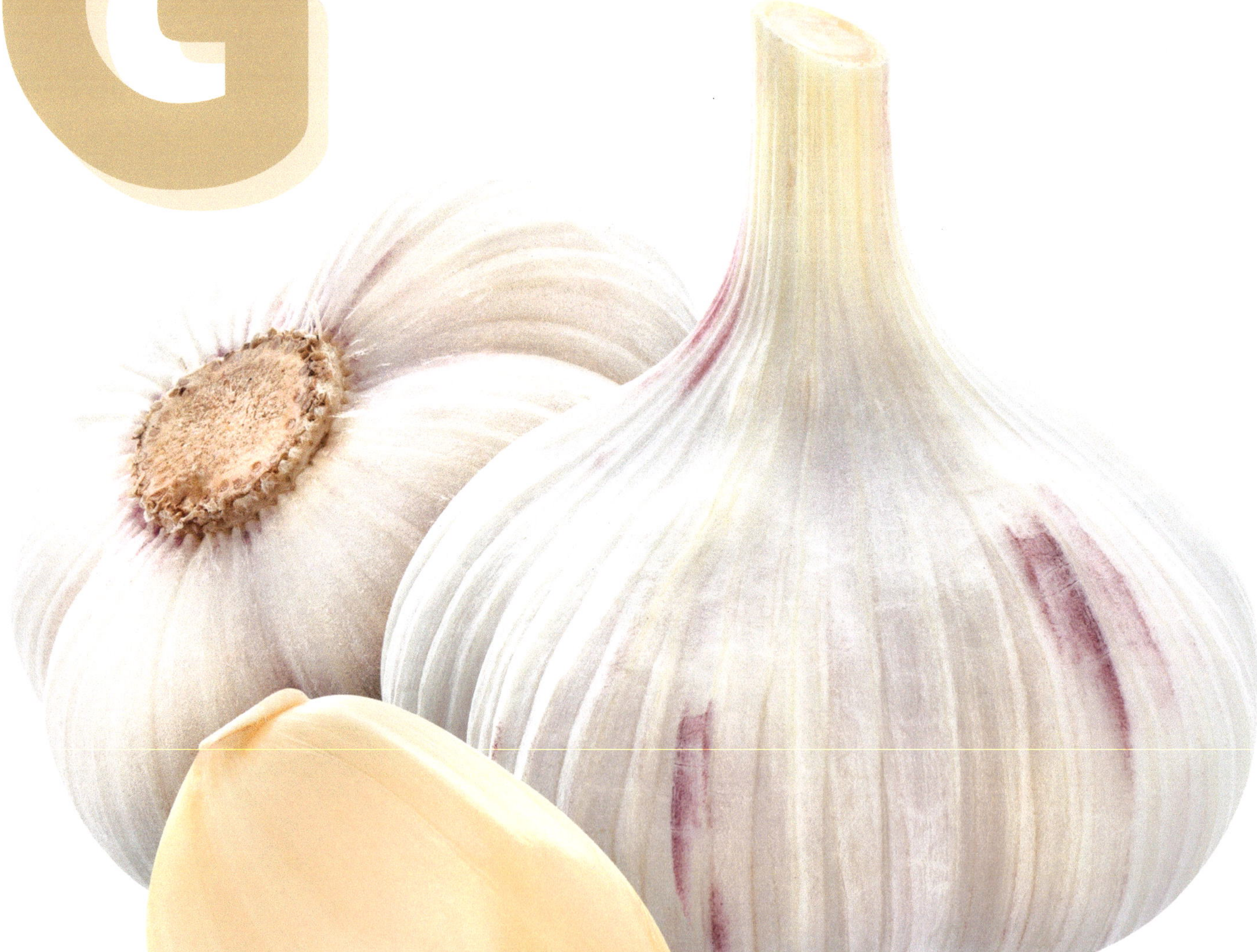

Garlic

Vegetable

g

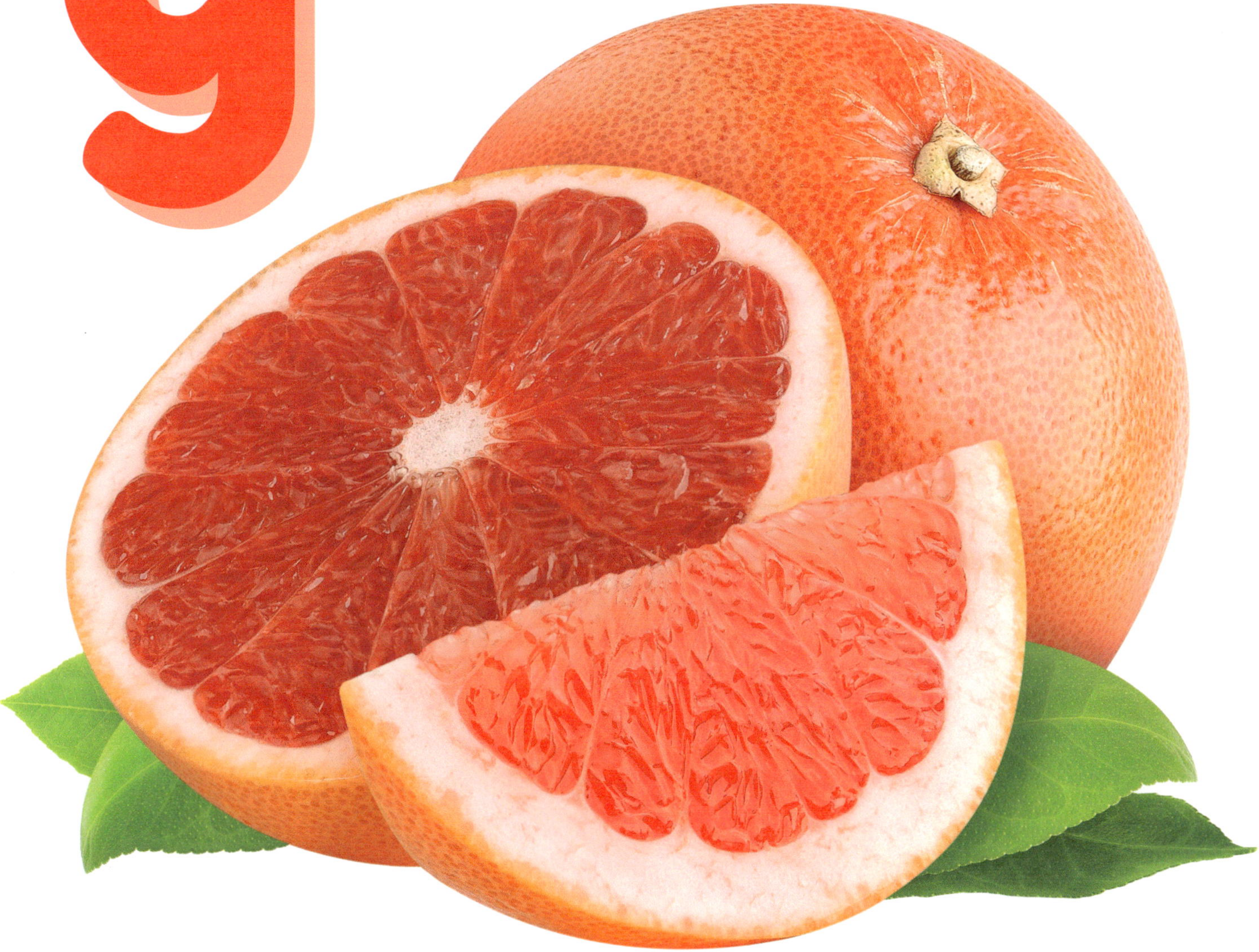

Fruit

Grapefruit

H

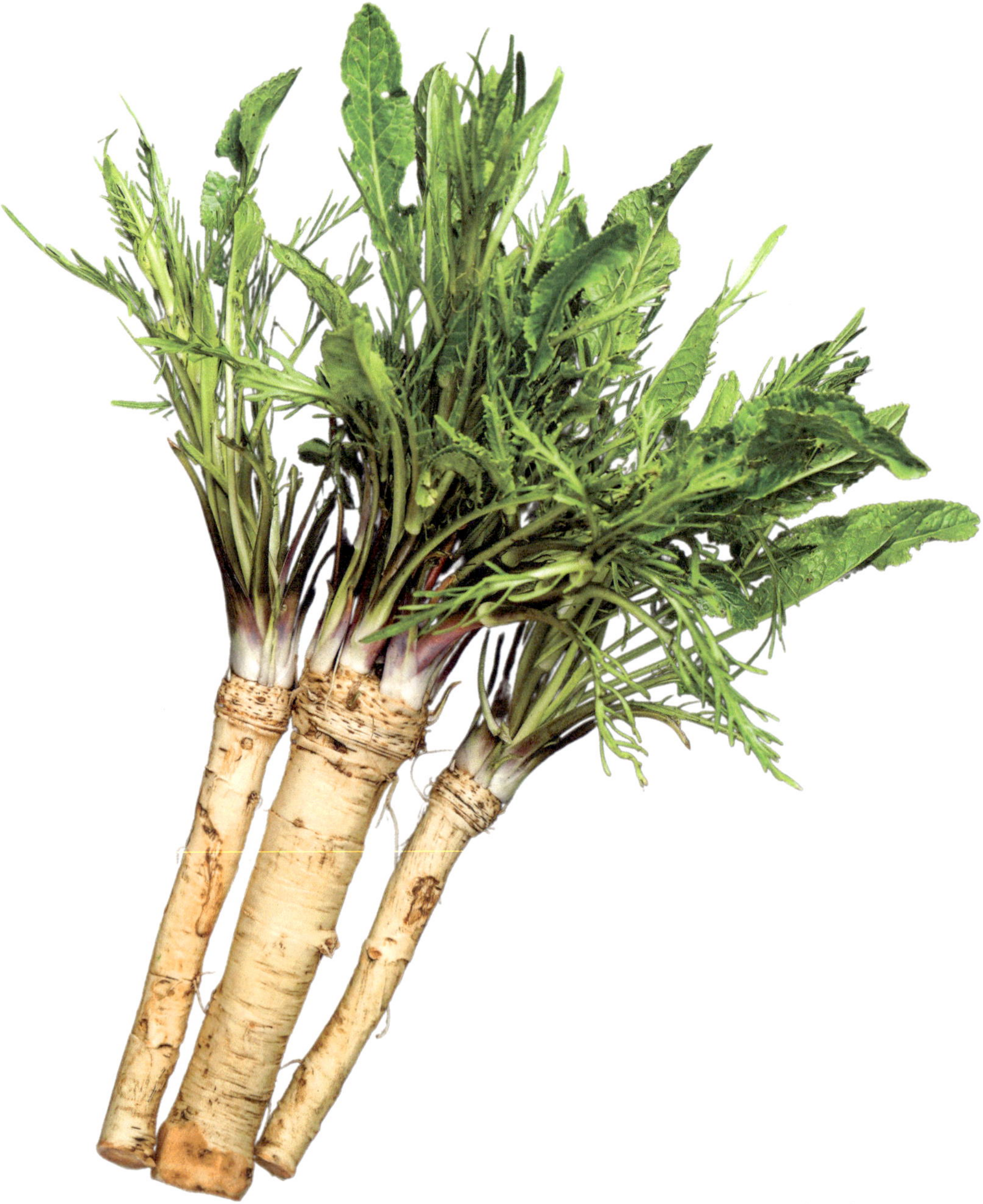

Horseradish

Vegetable

h

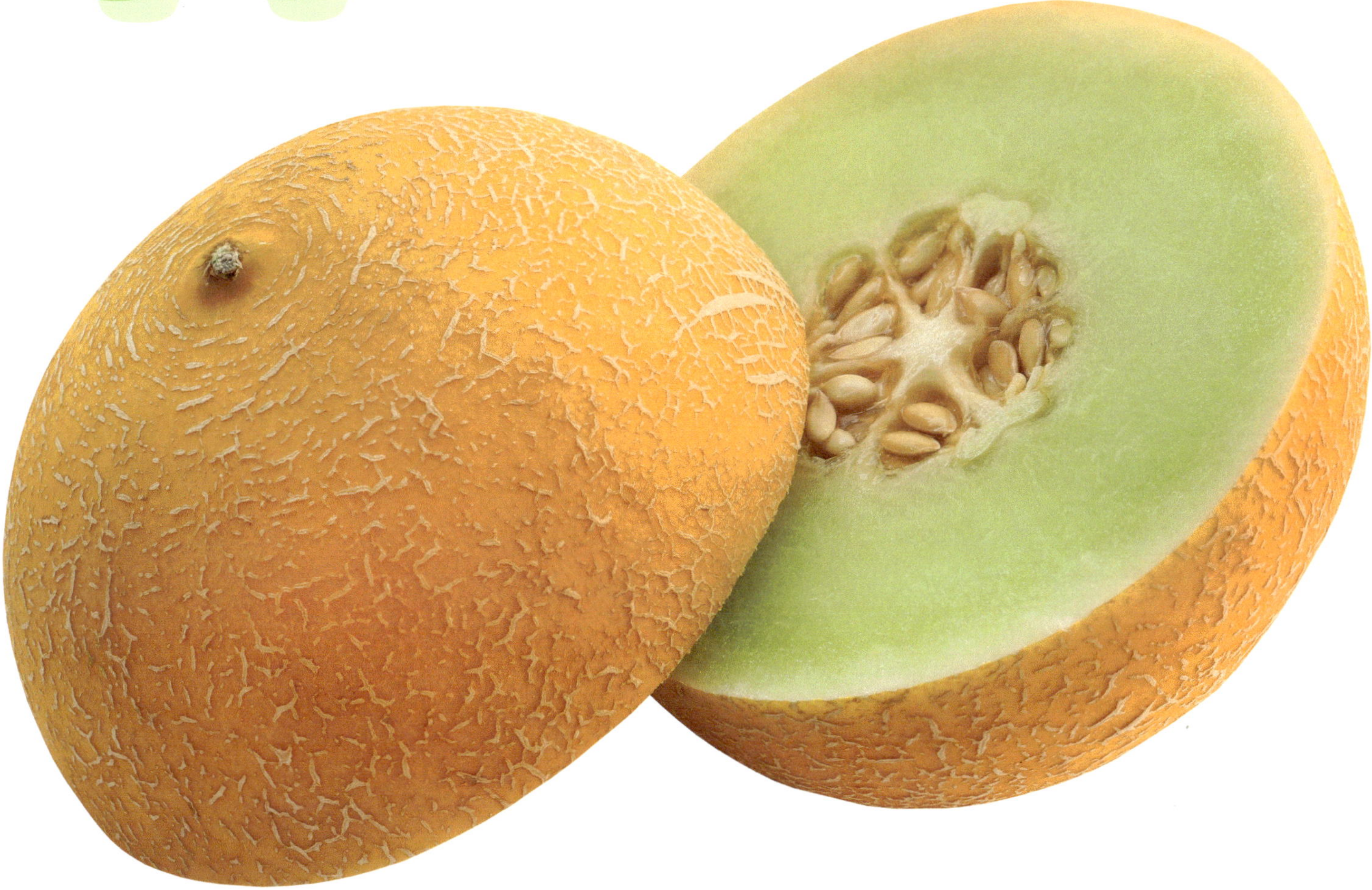

Fruit

Honeydew

I

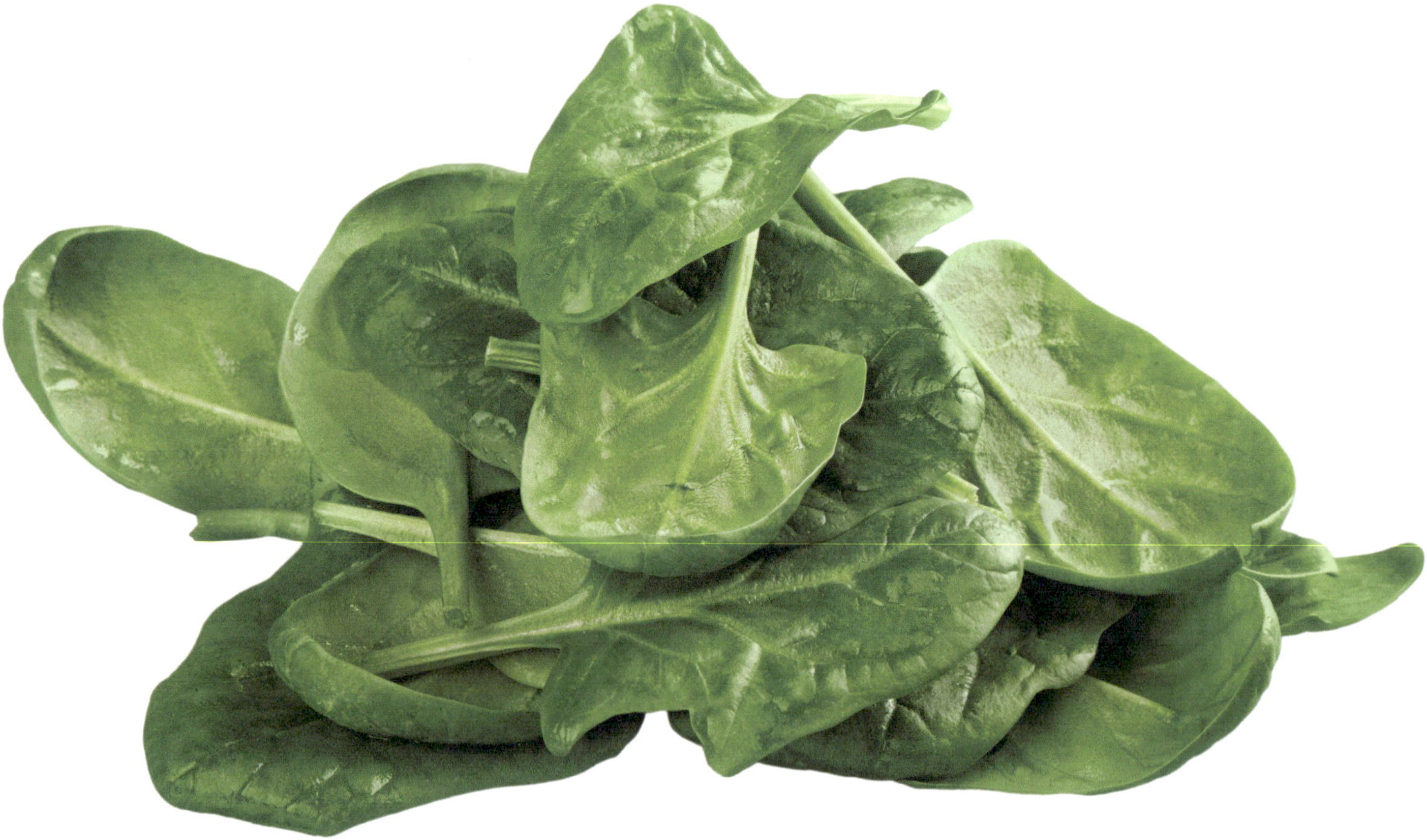

Spinach

Vegetable

i

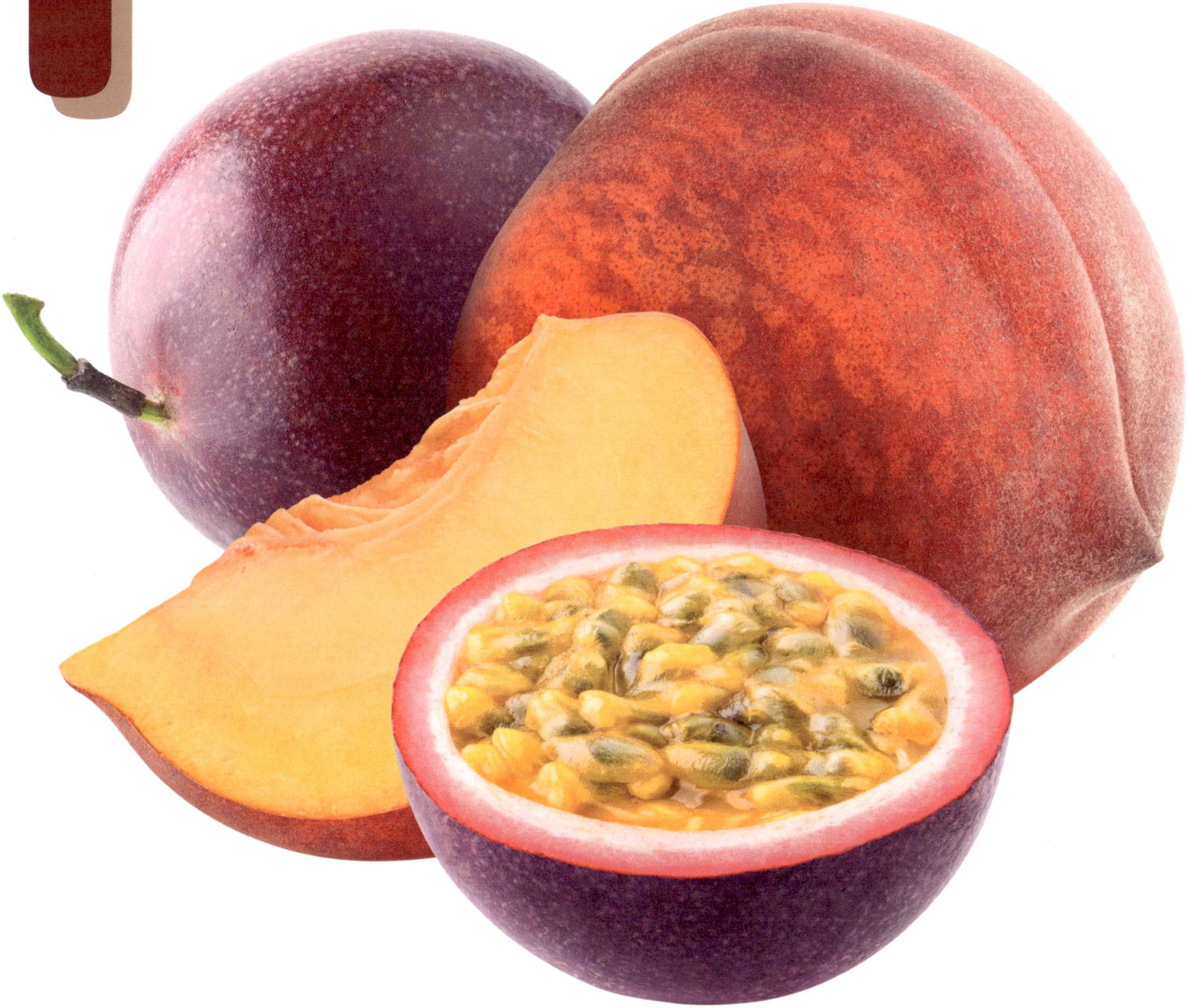

Fruit

Passionfruit

J

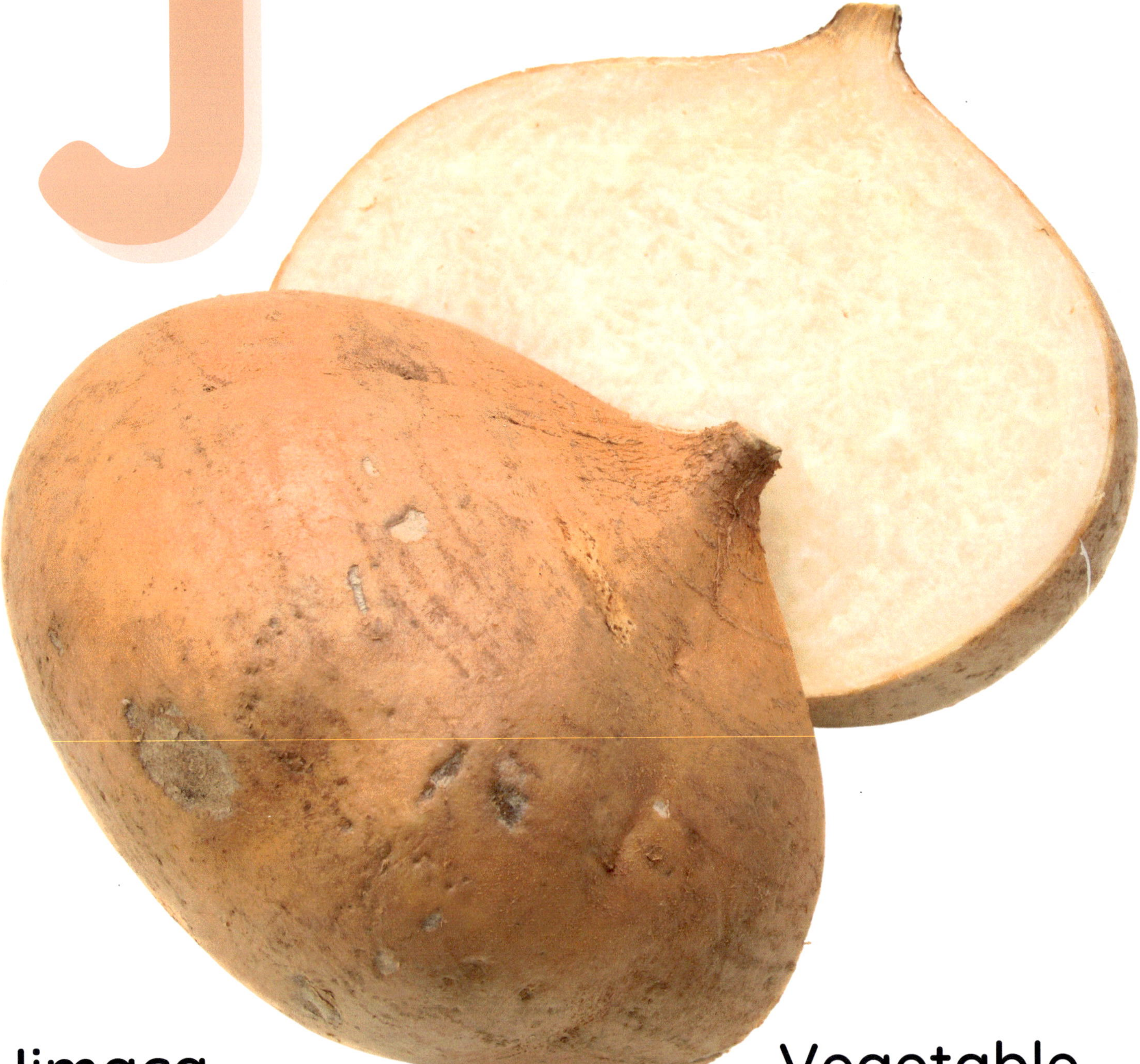

Jimaca

Vegetable

j

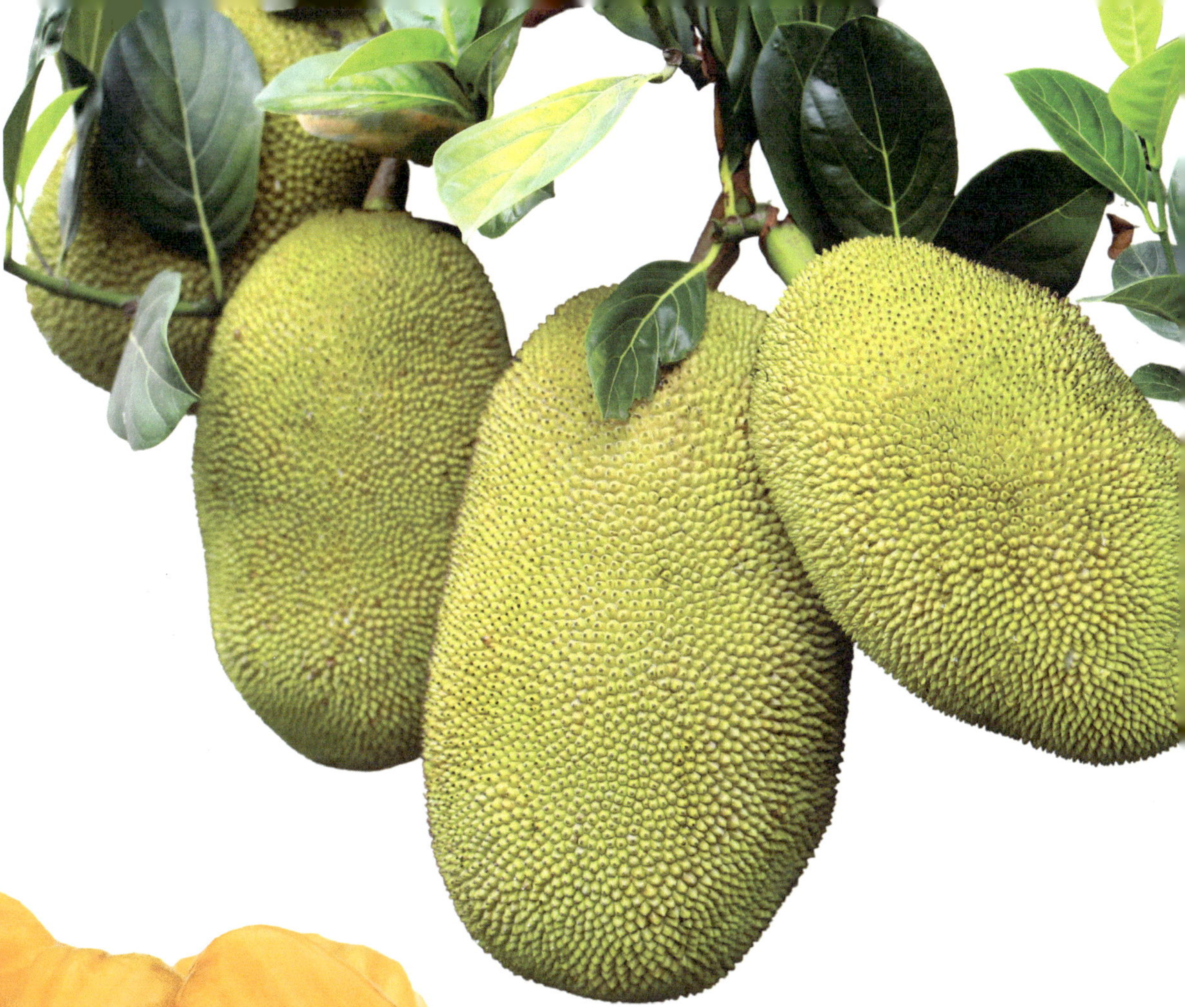

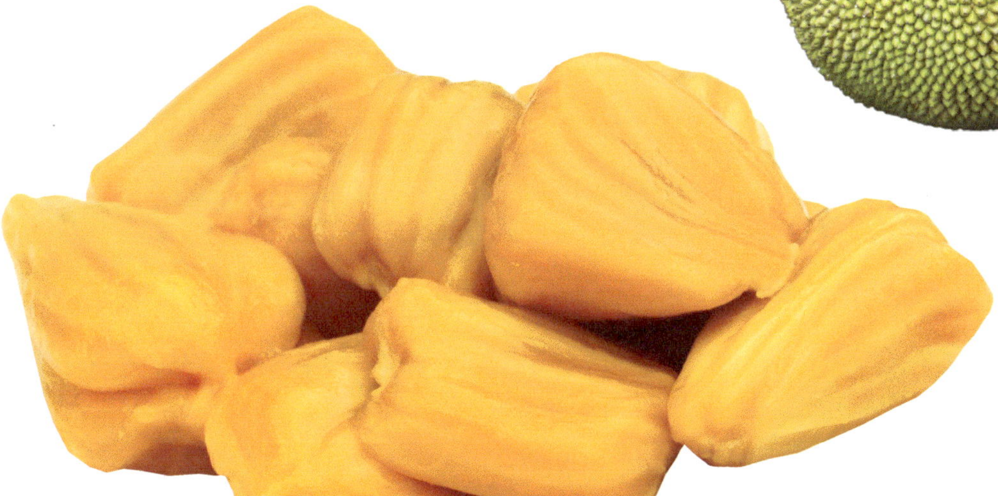

Fruit

Jackfruit

K

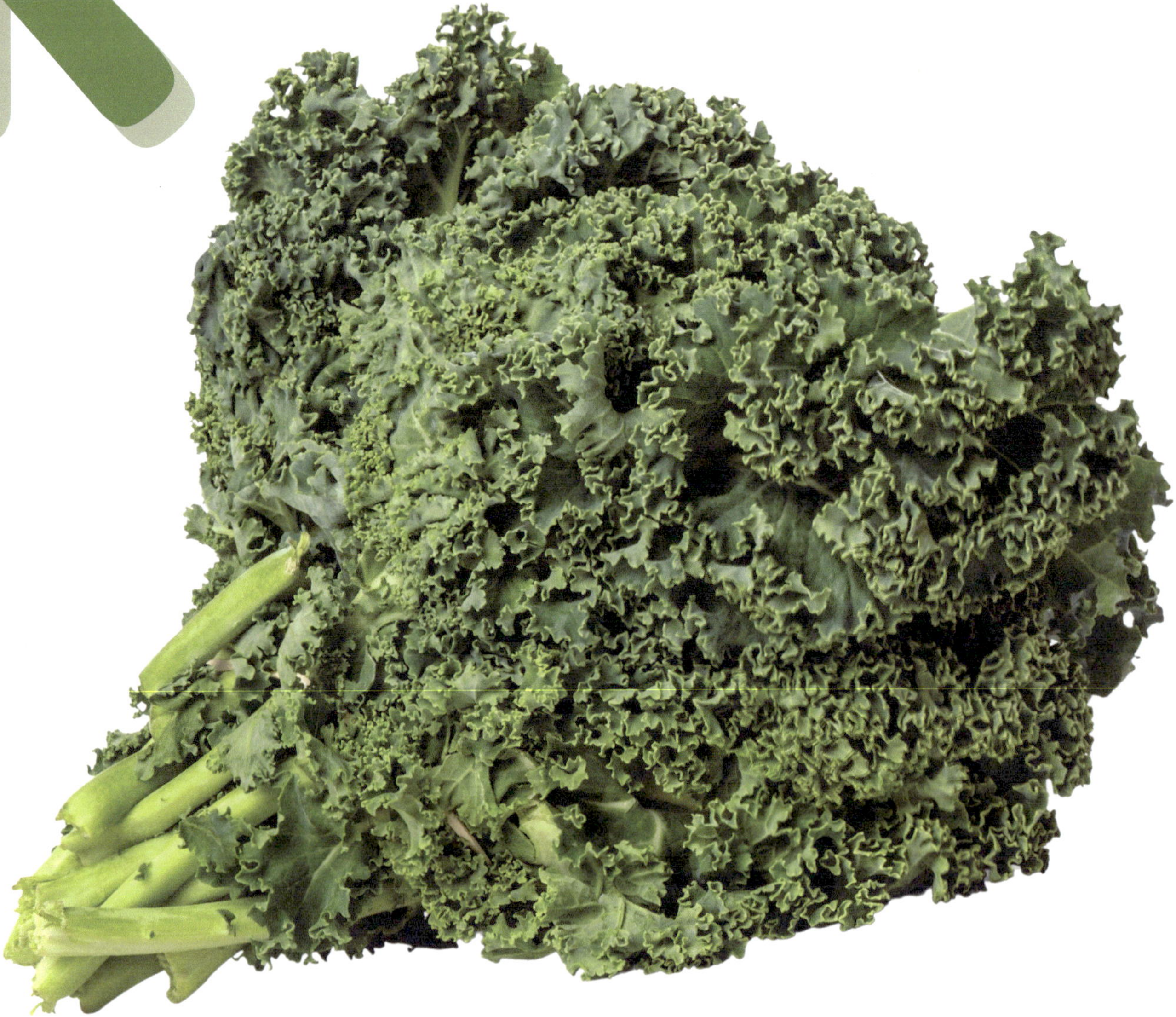

Kale

Vegetable

k

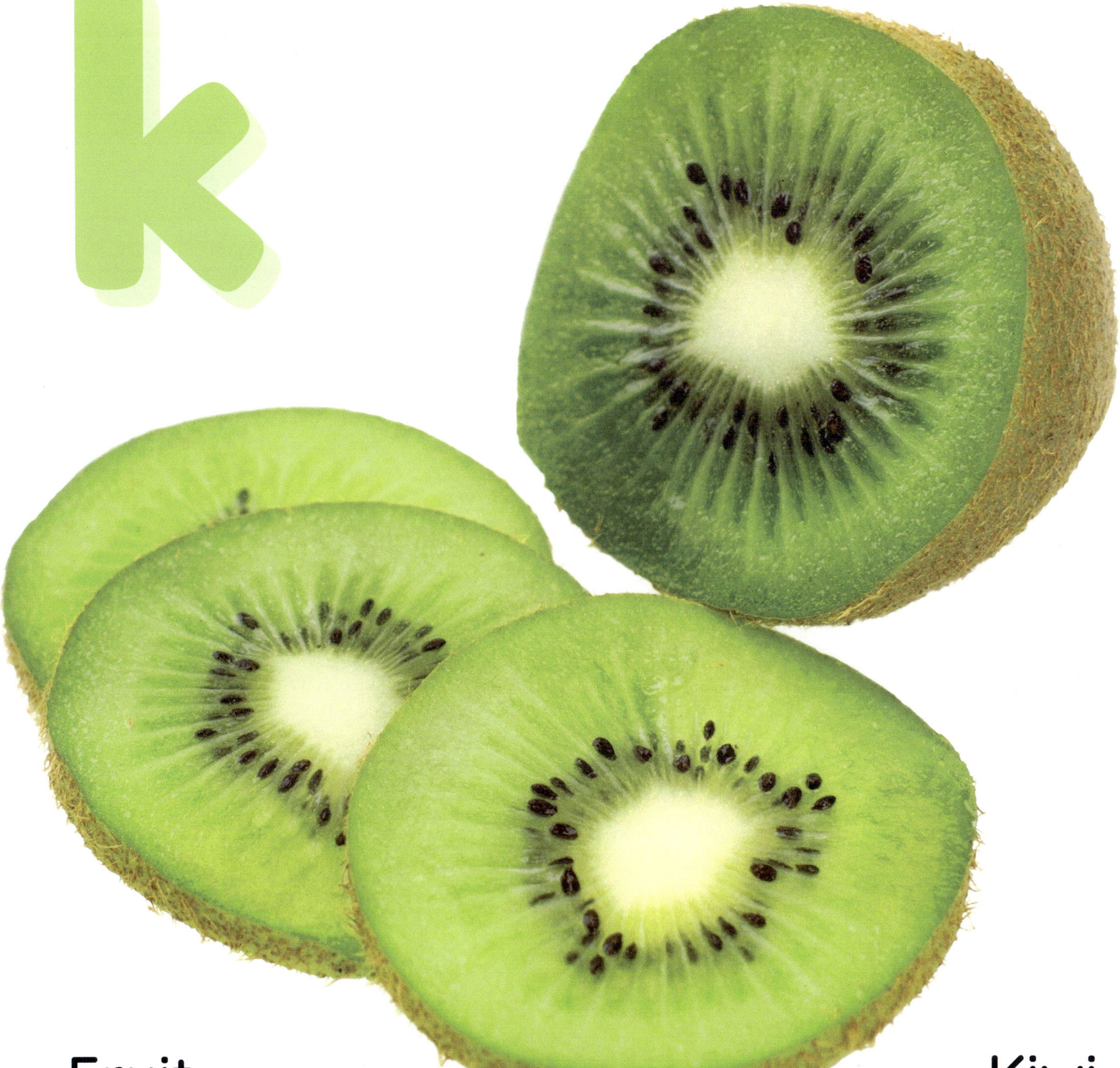

Fruit

Kiwi

L

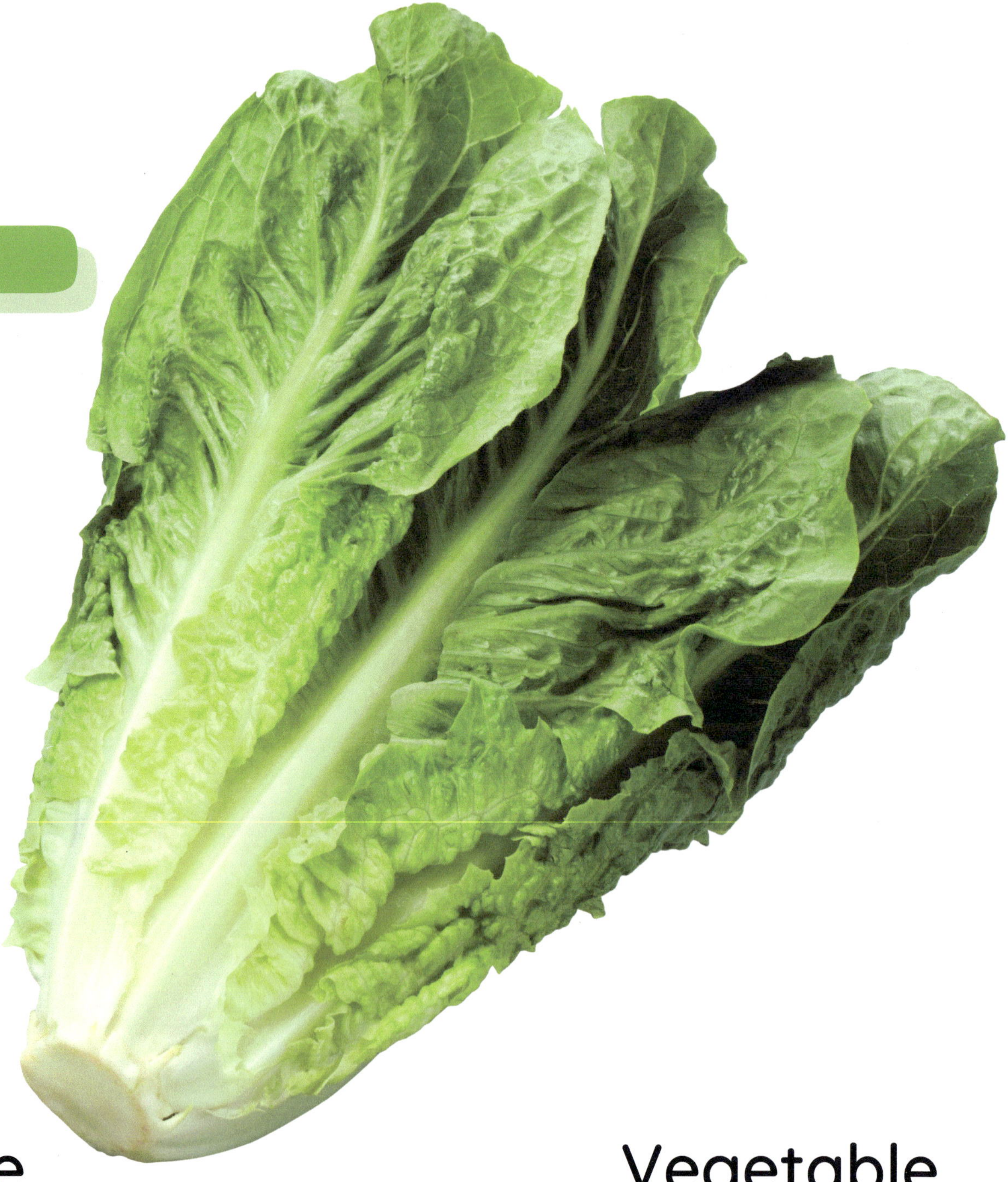

Lettuce

Vegetable

l

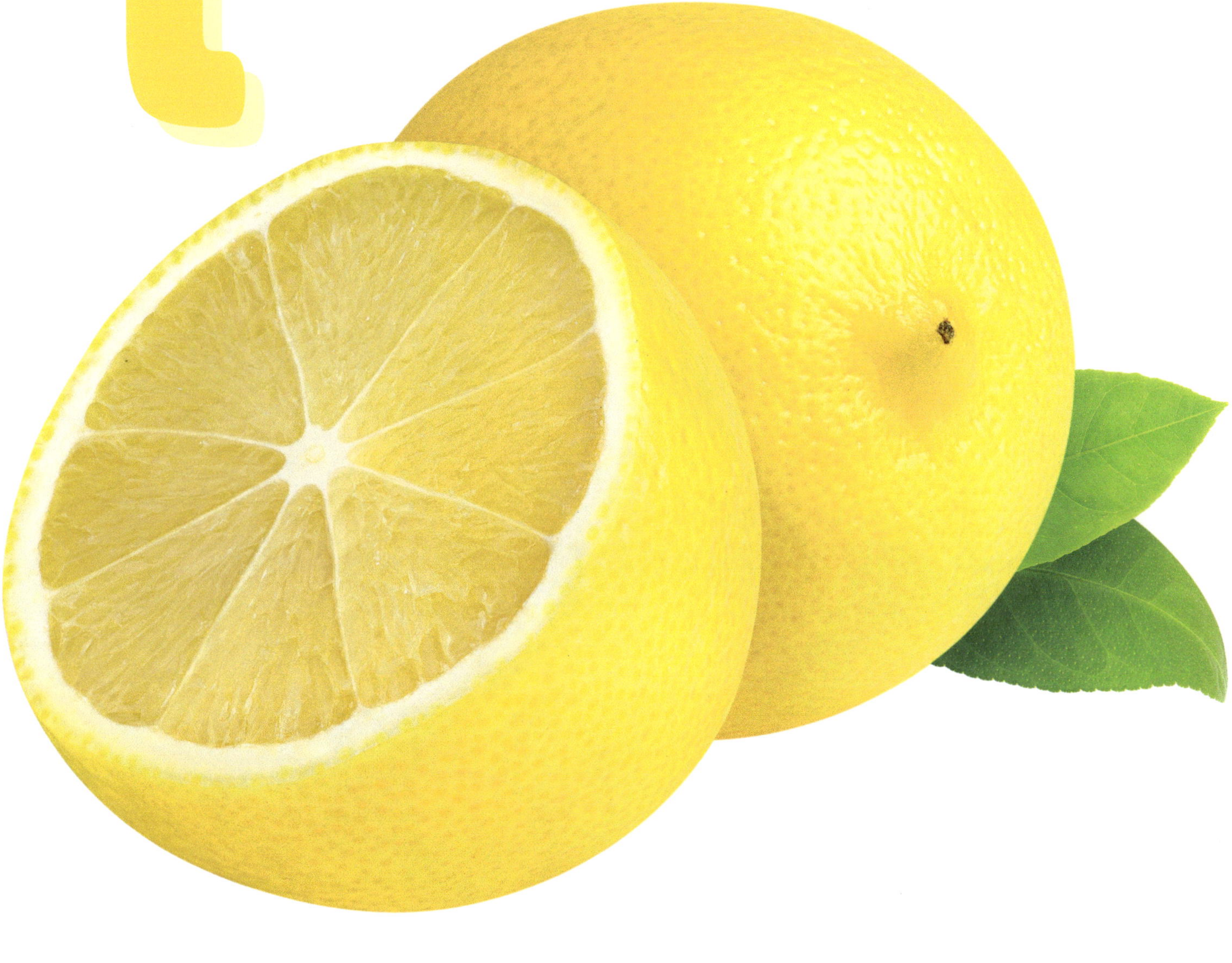

Fruit

Lemon

M

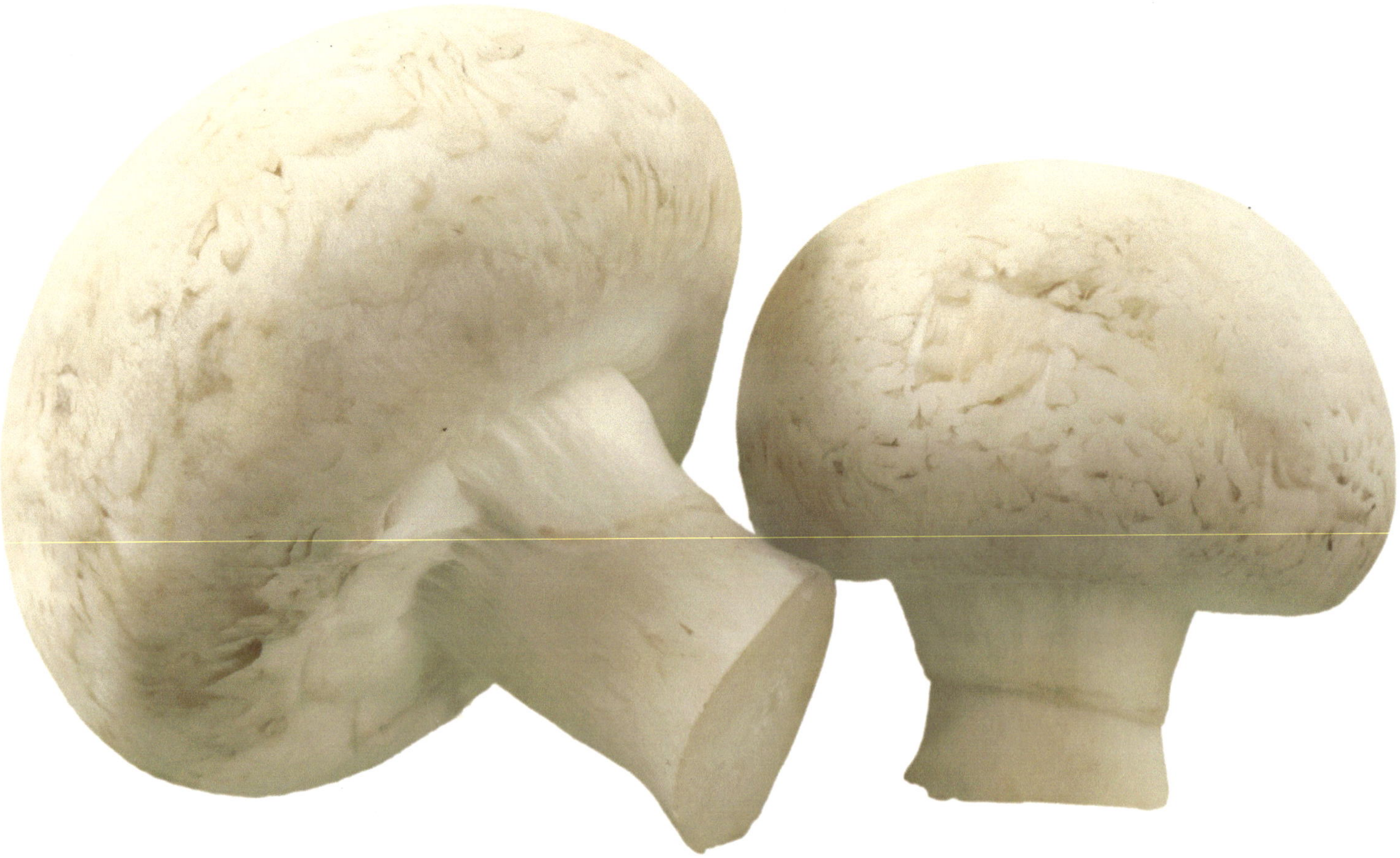

Mushroom

Vegetable

m

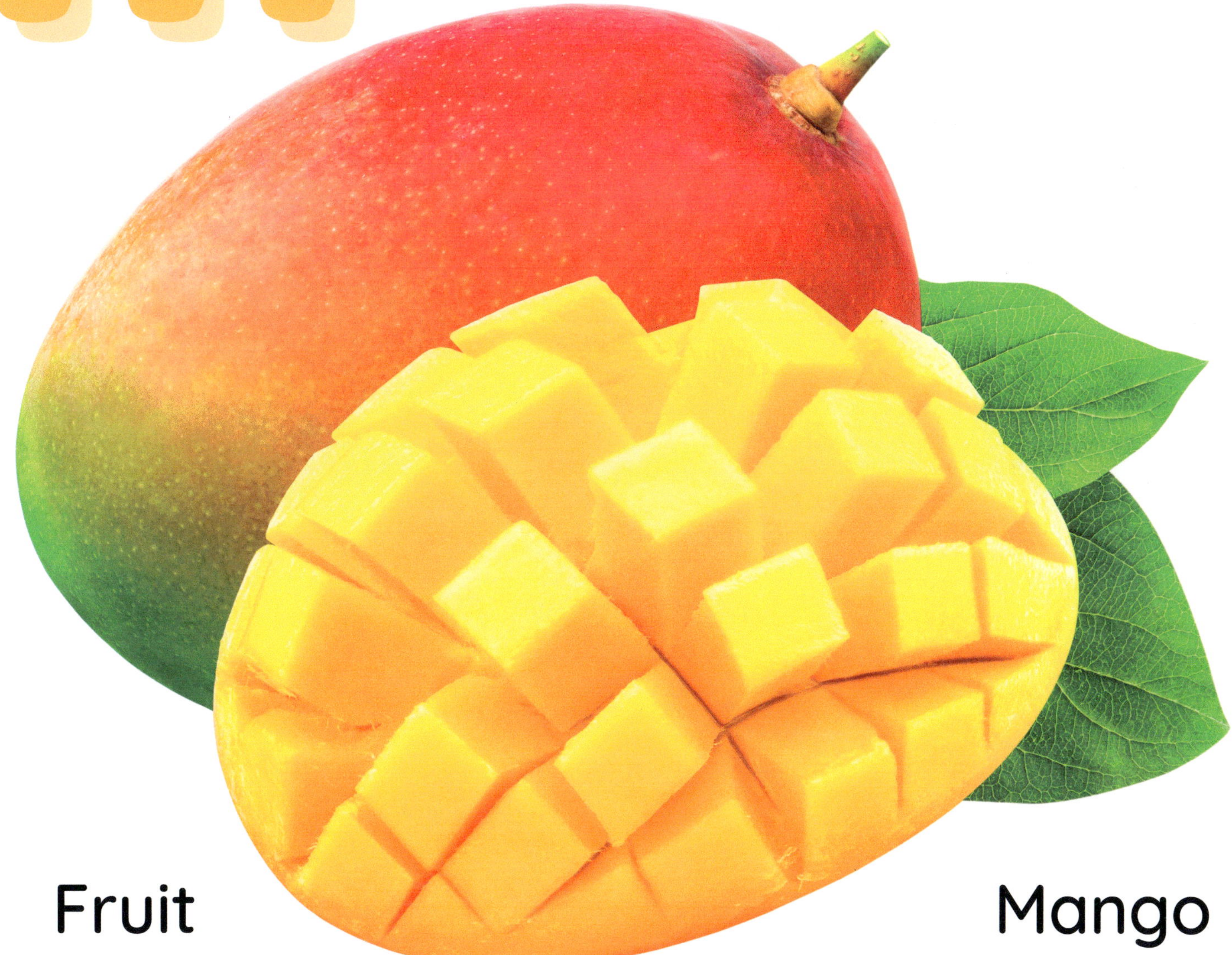

Fruit

Mango

N

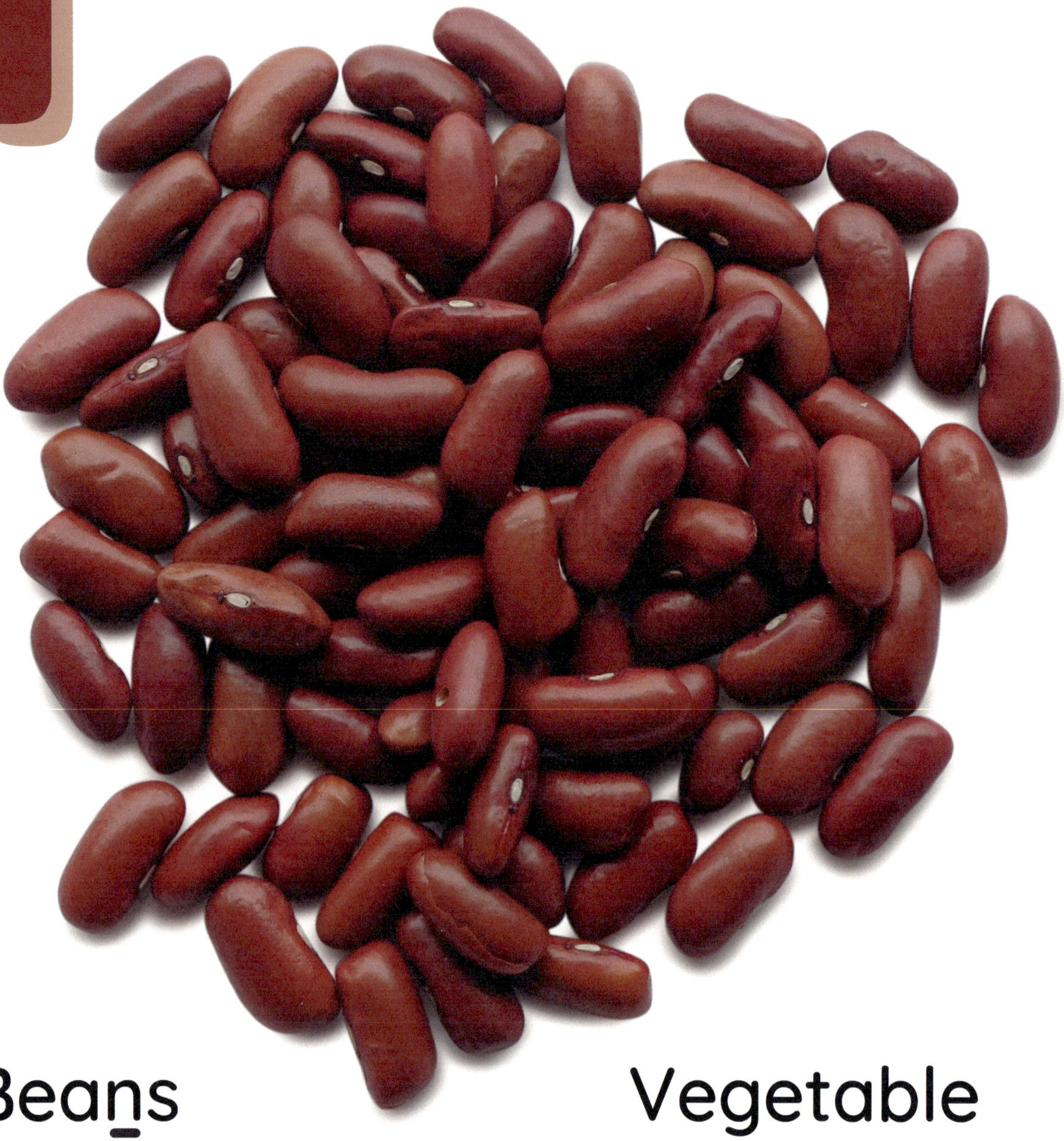

Kidney Beans

Vegetable

n

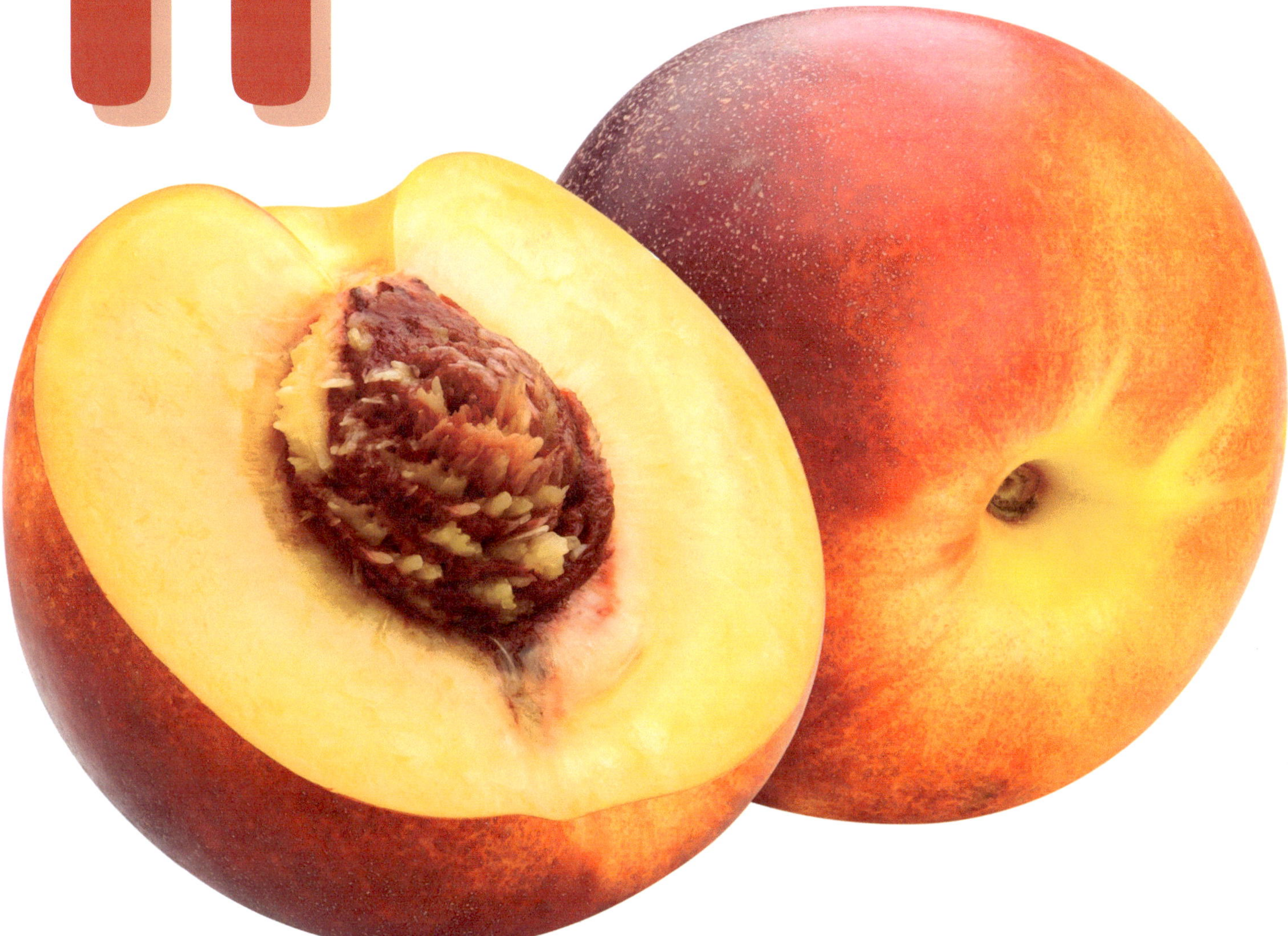

Fruit

Nectarine

O

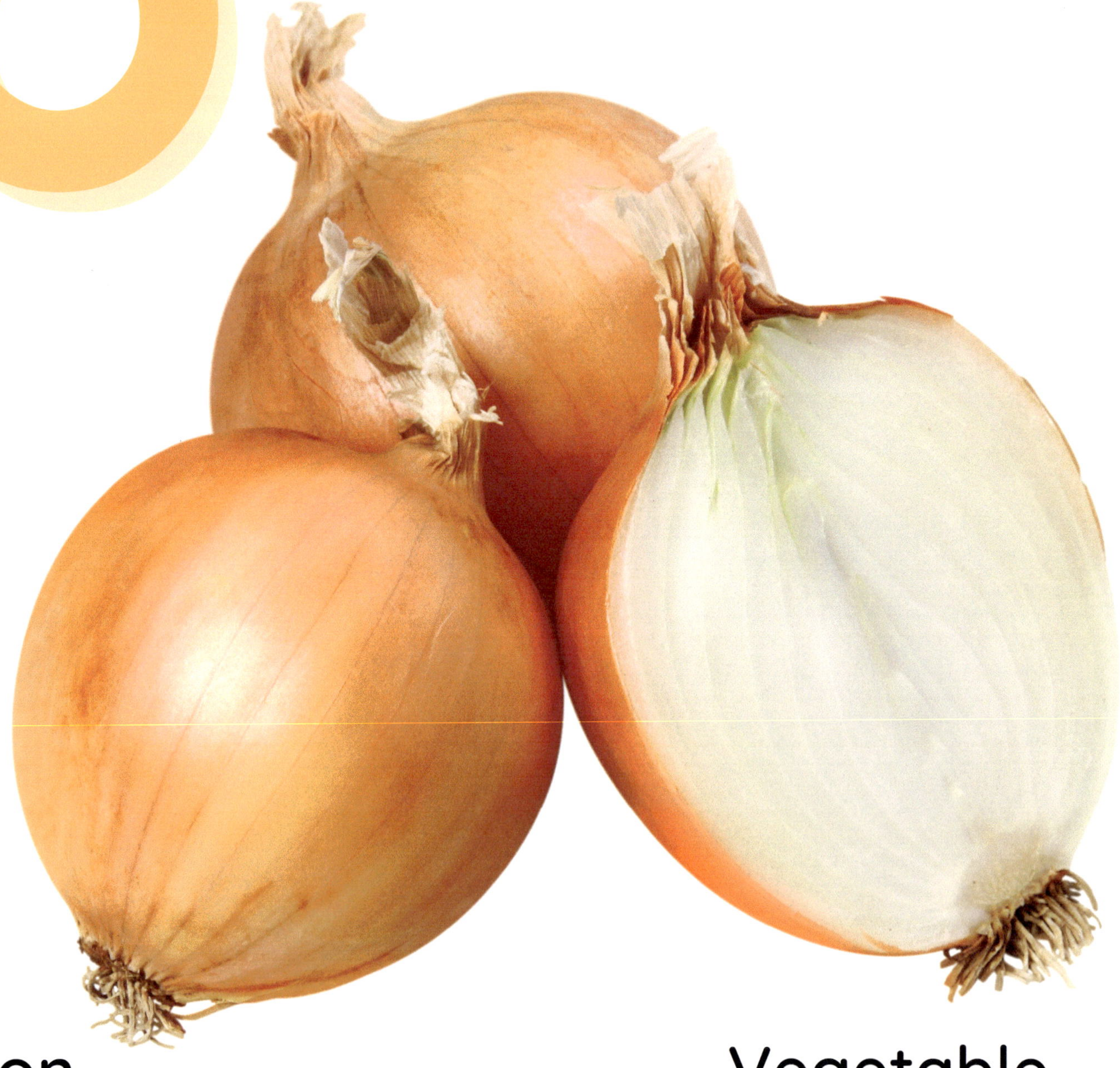

Onion

Vegetable

O

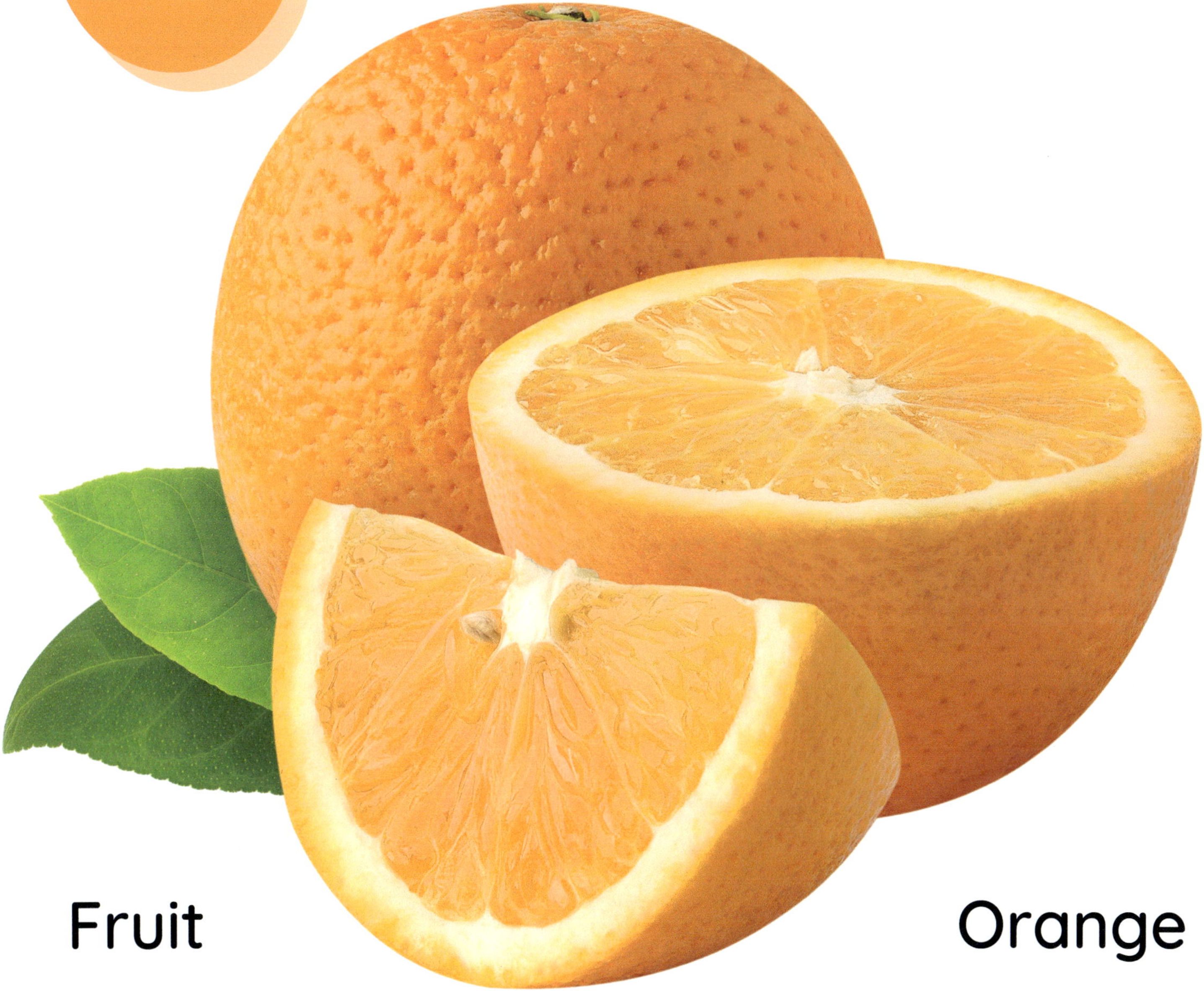

Fruit

Orange

P

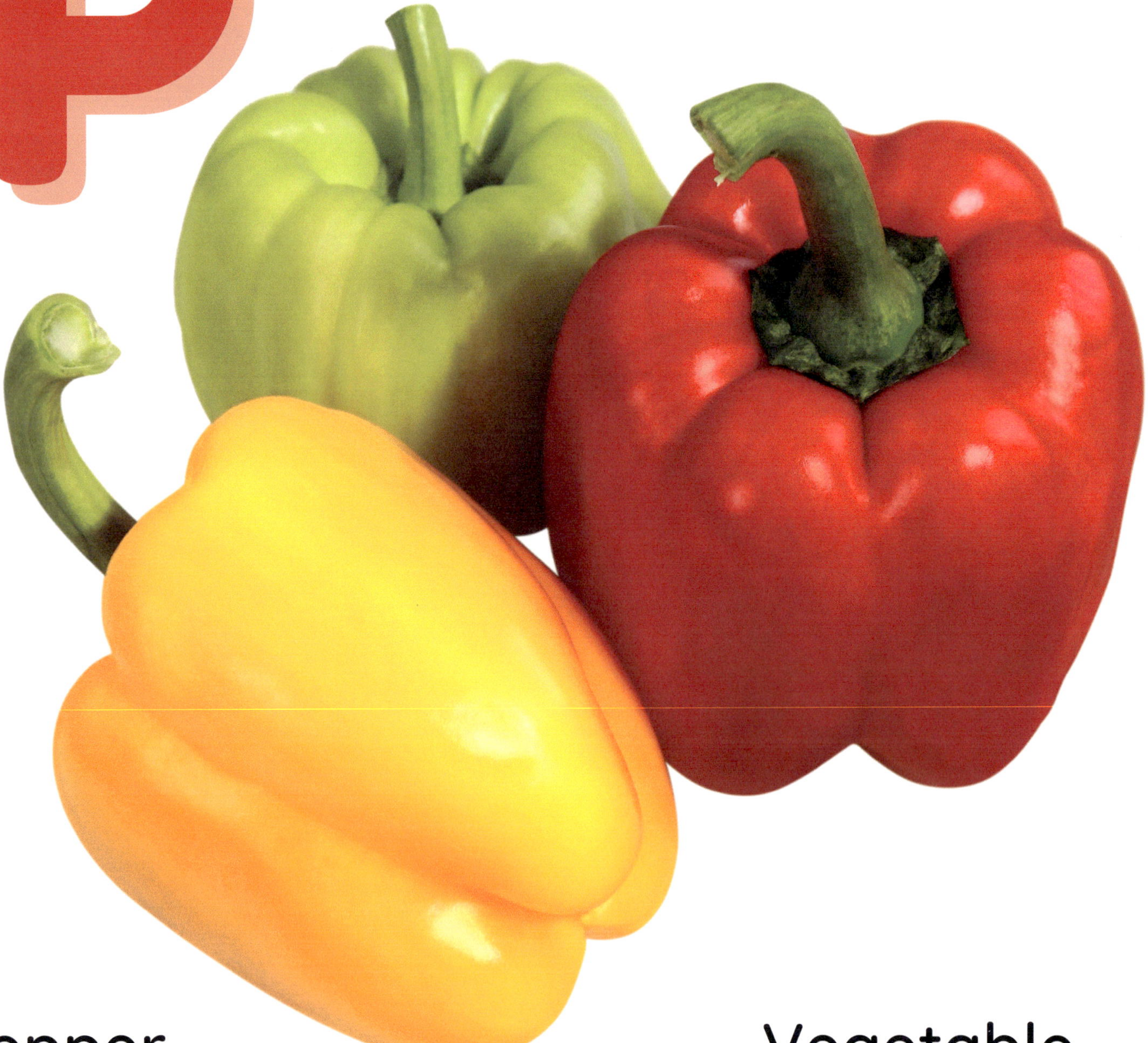

Pepper

Vegetable

p

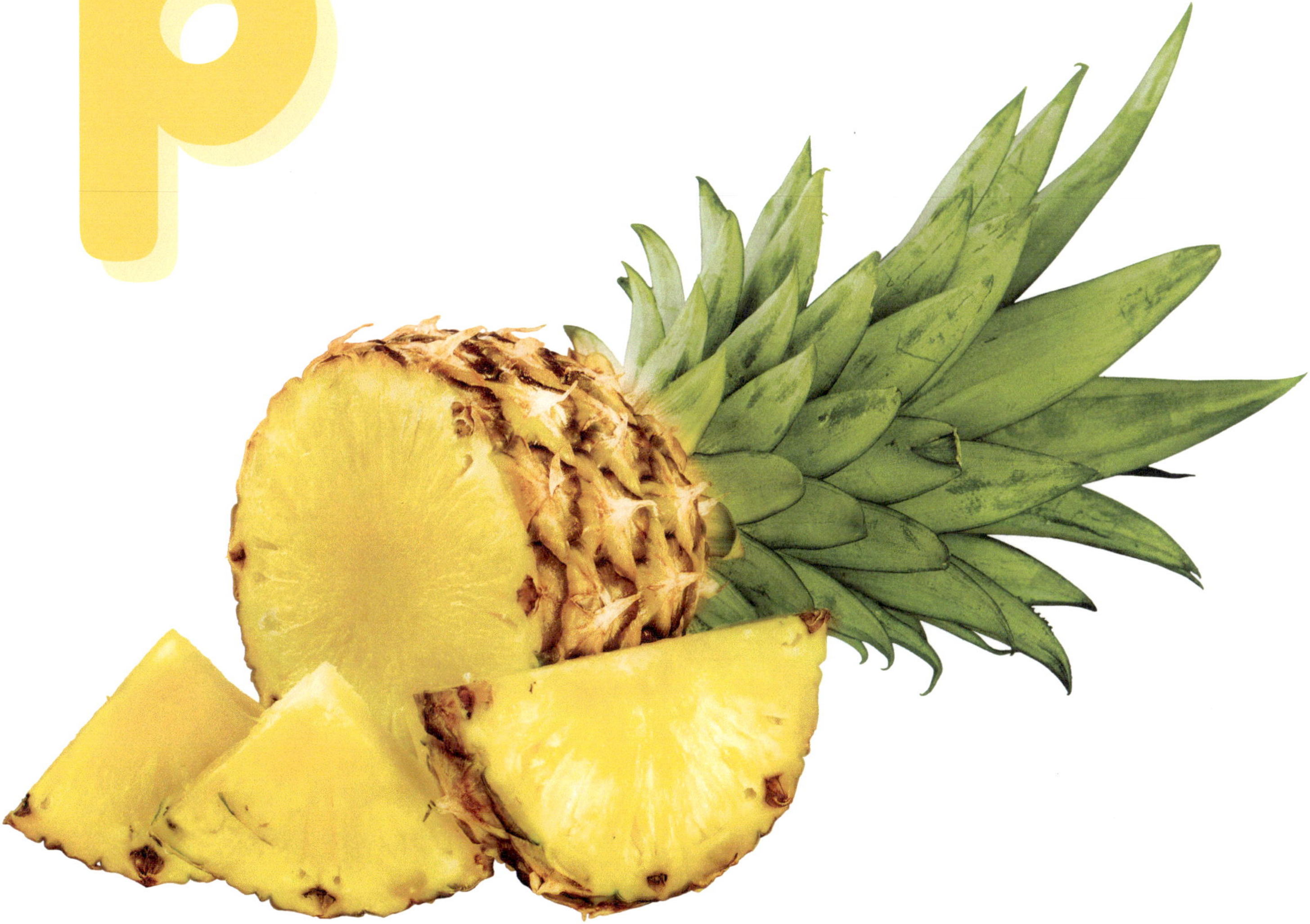

Fruit

Pineapple

Q

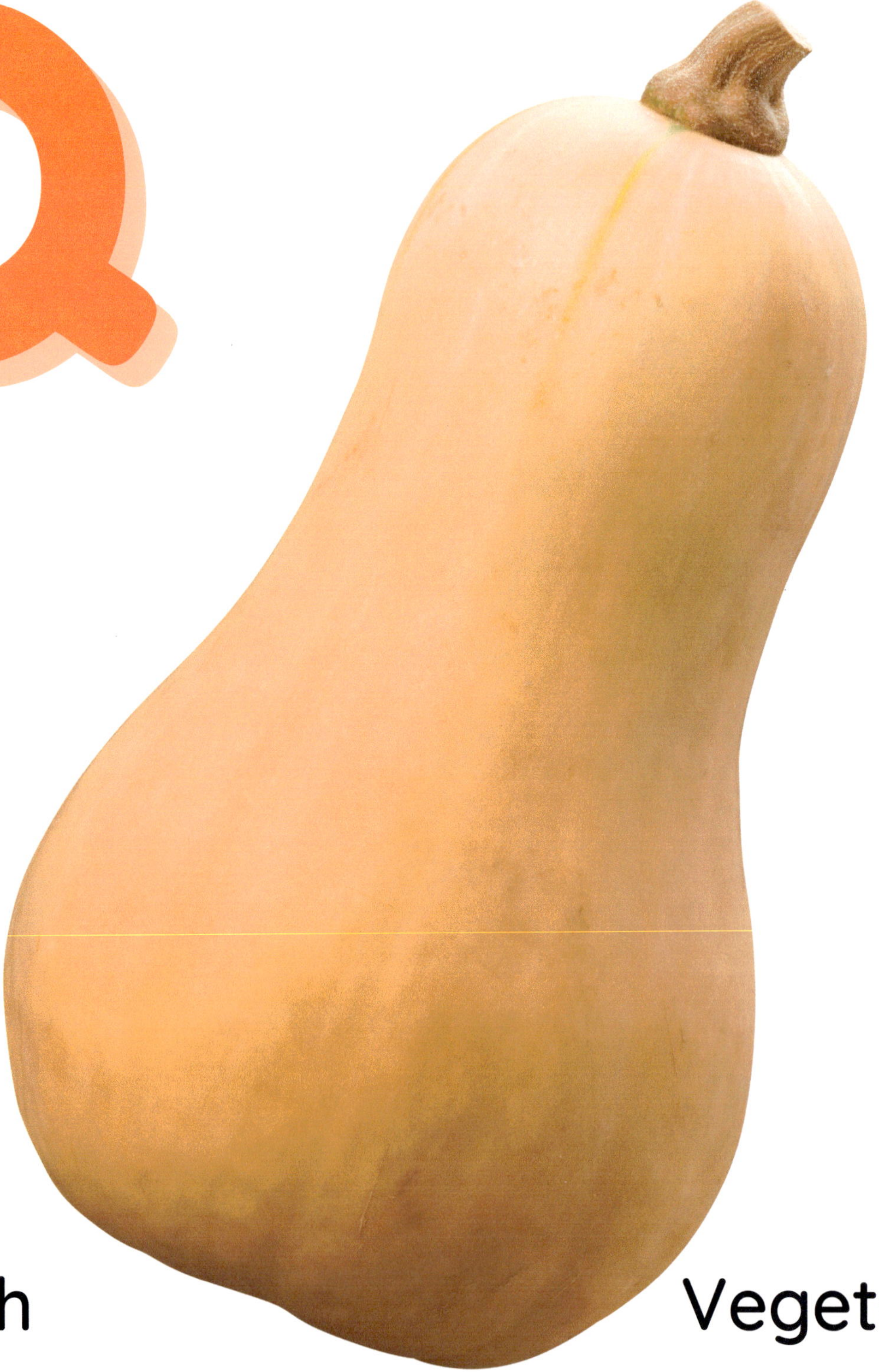

Squash

Vegetable

q

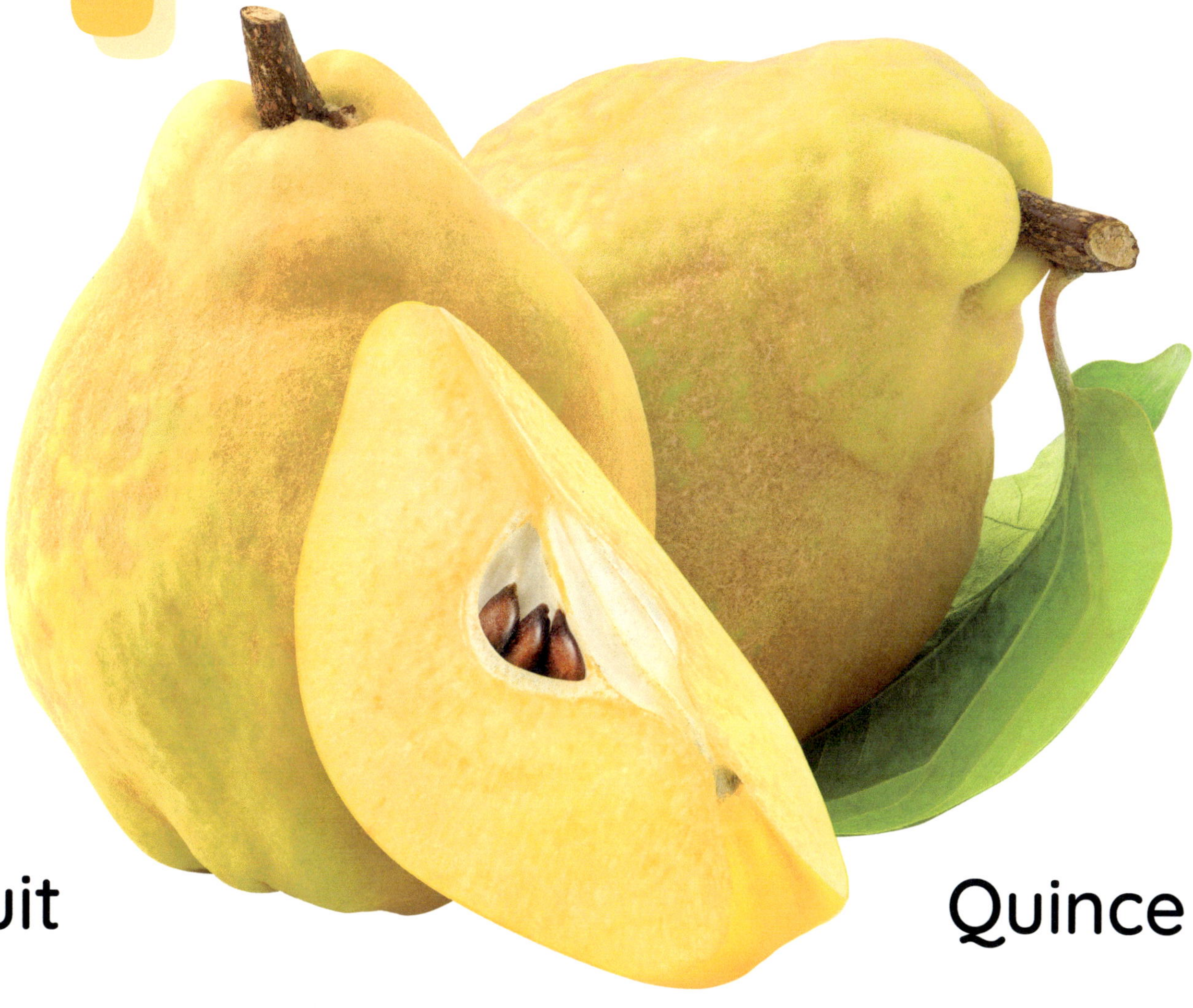

Fruit

Quince

R

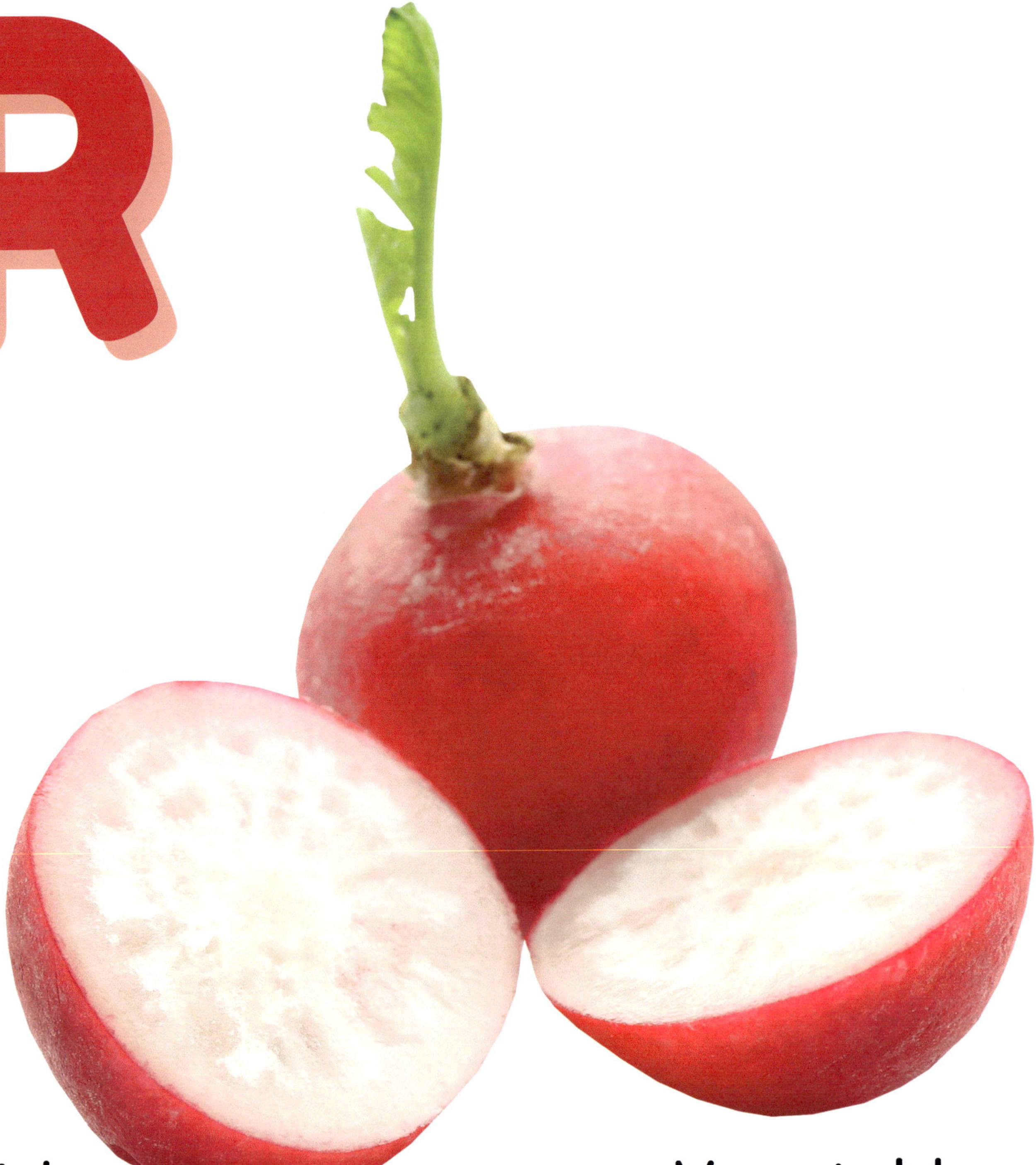

Radish

Vegetable

r

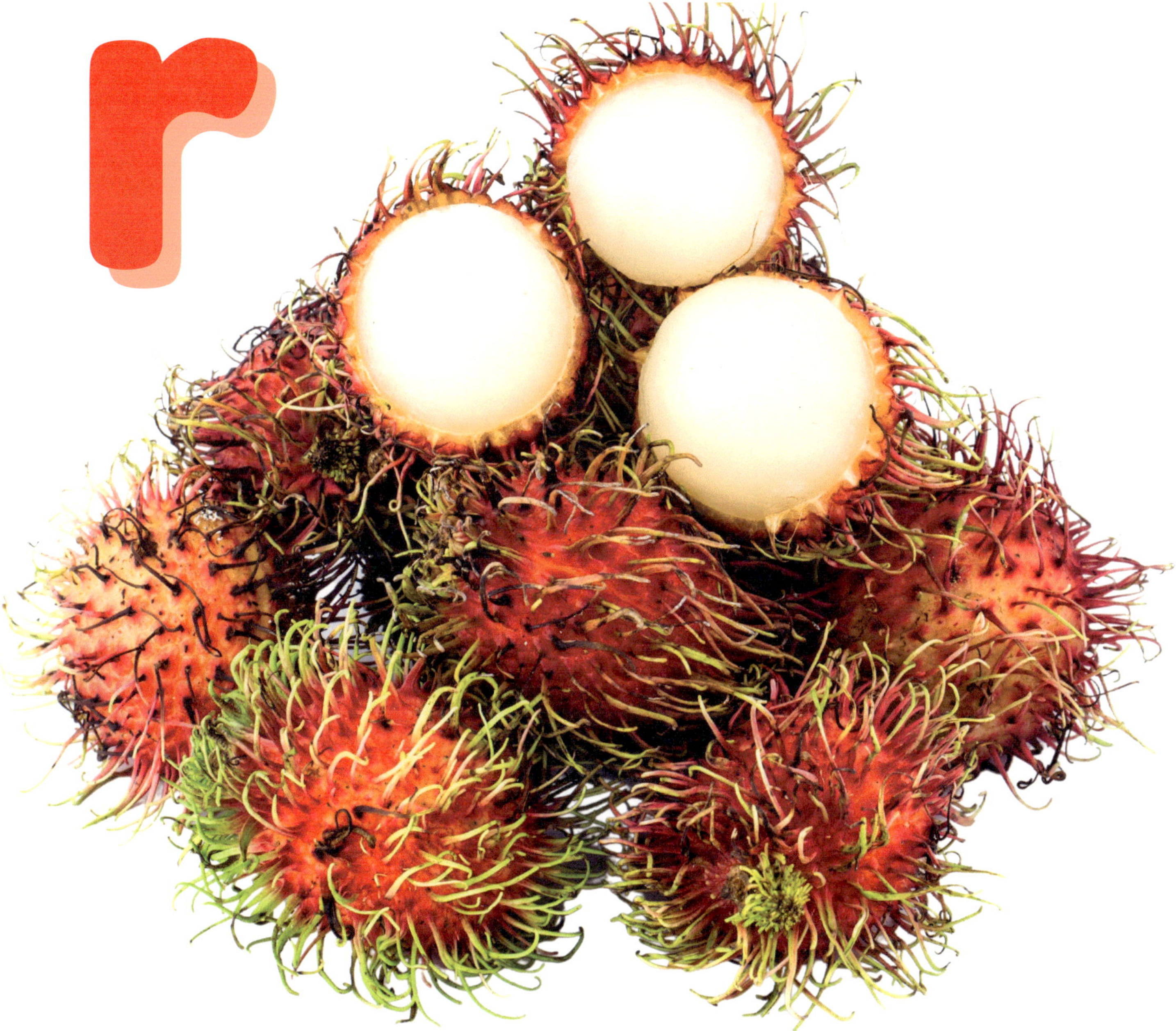

Fruit

Rambutan

S

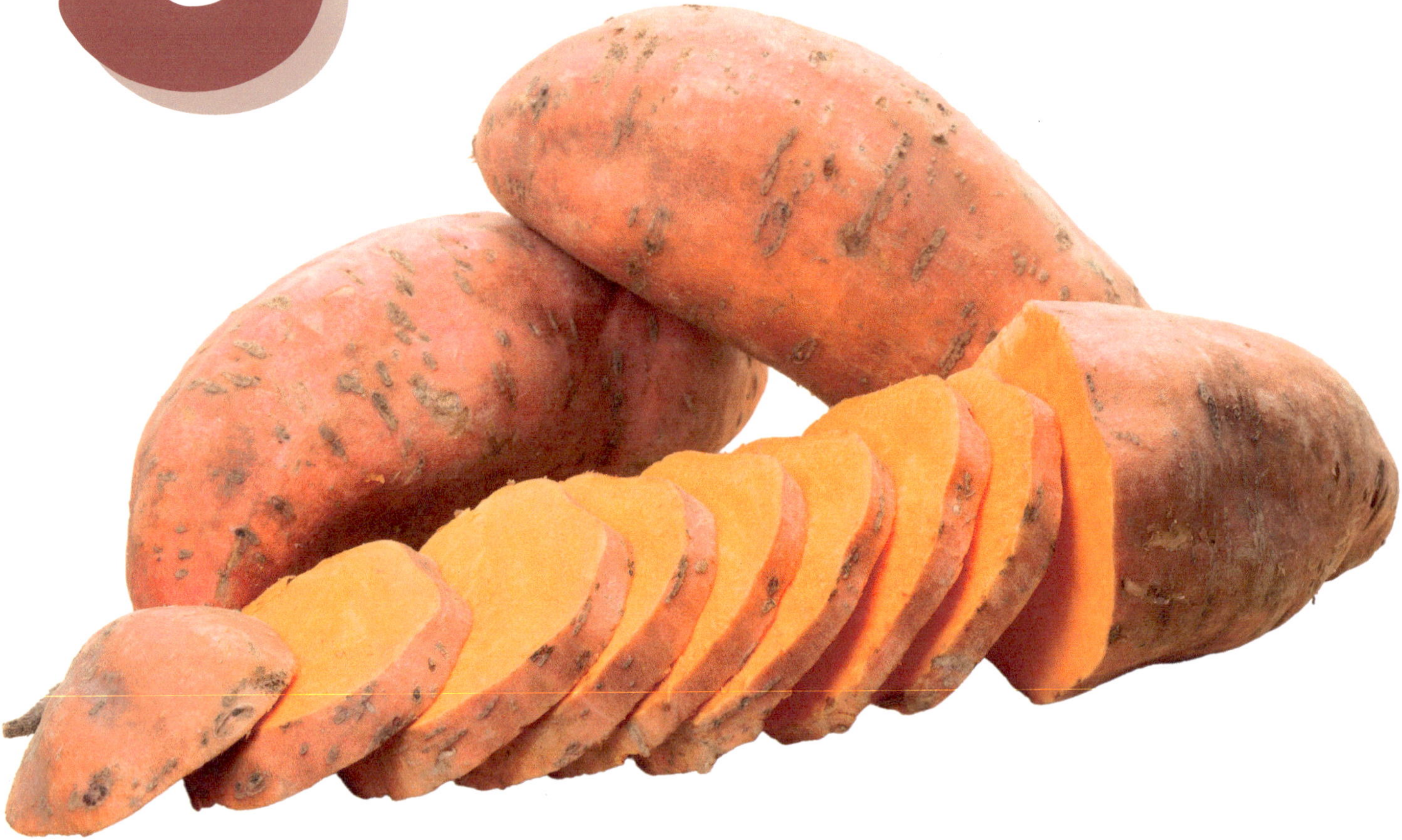

Sweet Potato

Vegetable

S

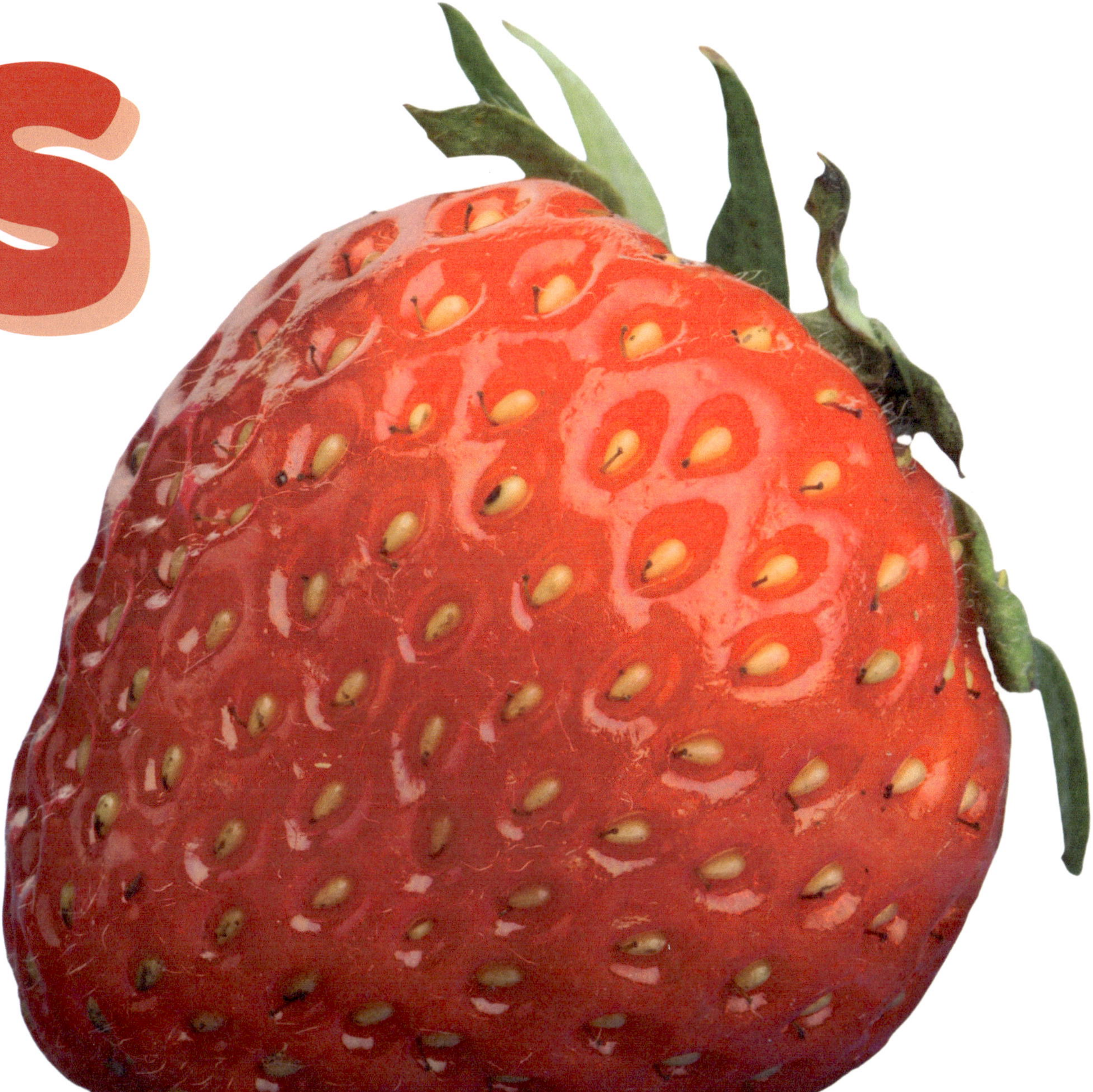

Fruit

Strawberry

T

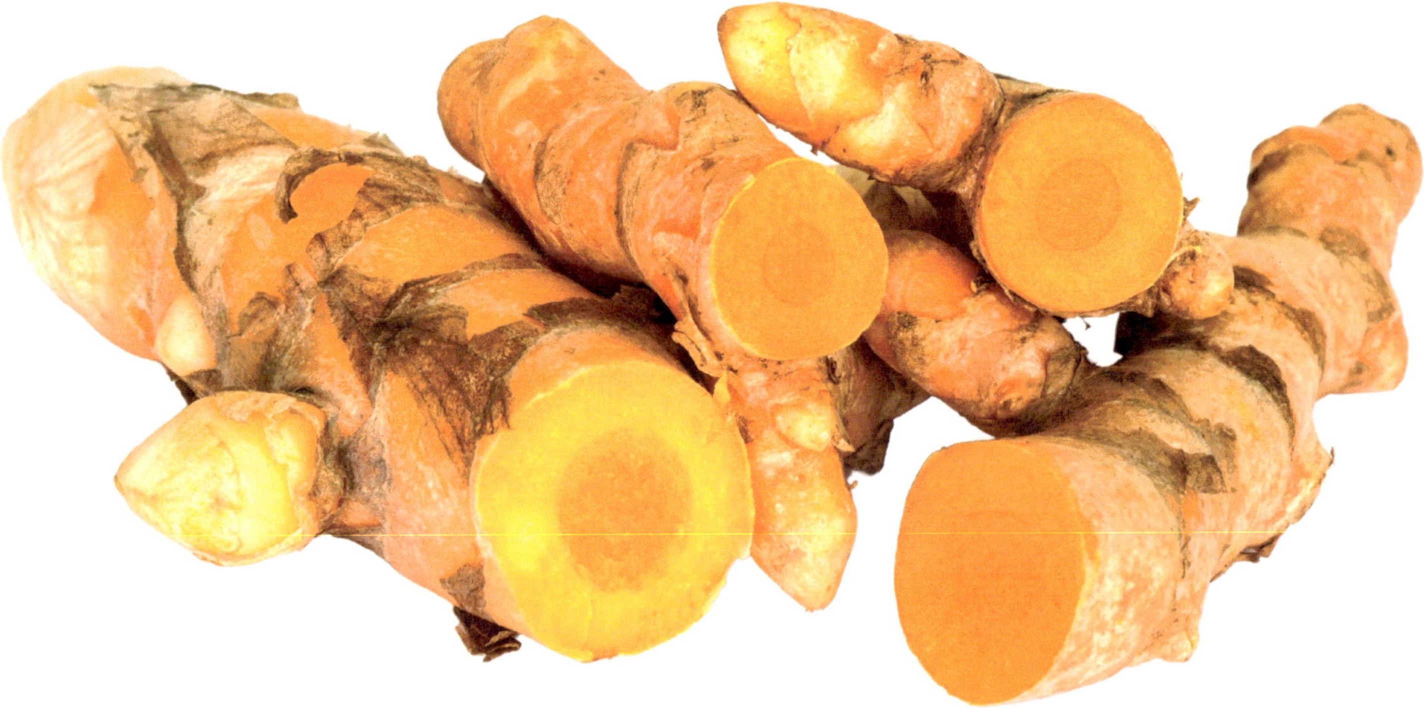

Tumeric

Vegetable

t

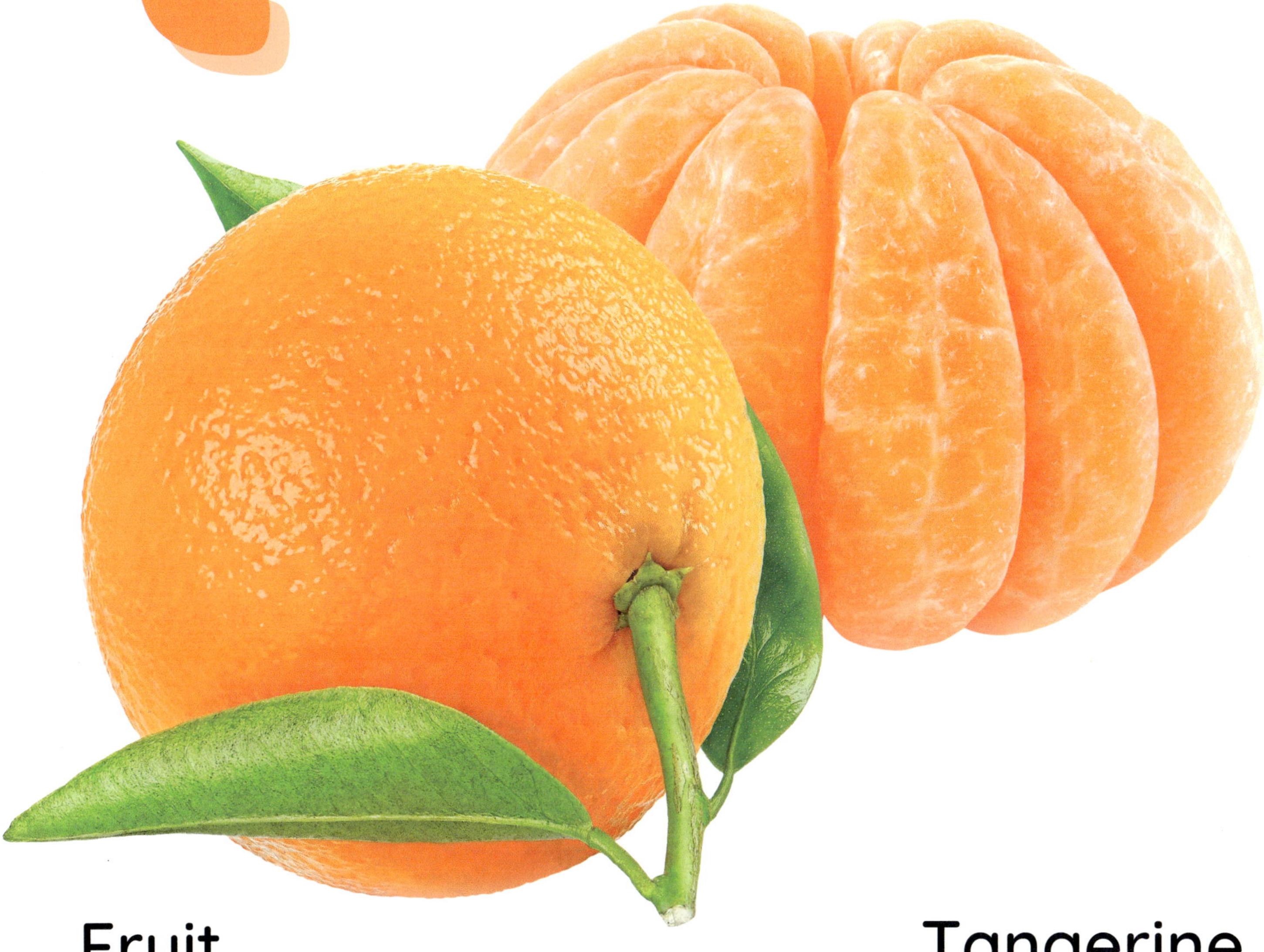

Fruit

Tangerine

U

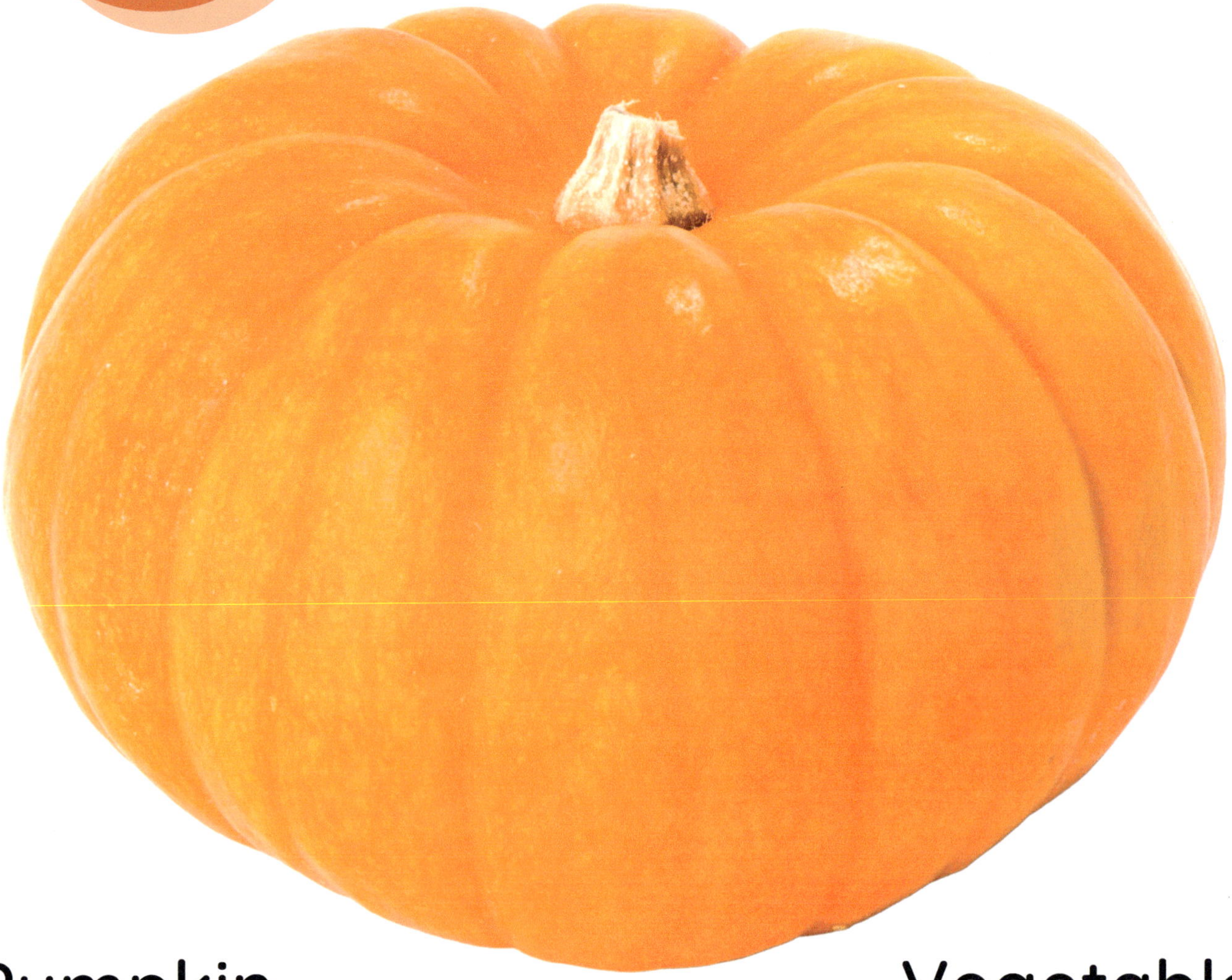

Pumpkin

Vegetable

u

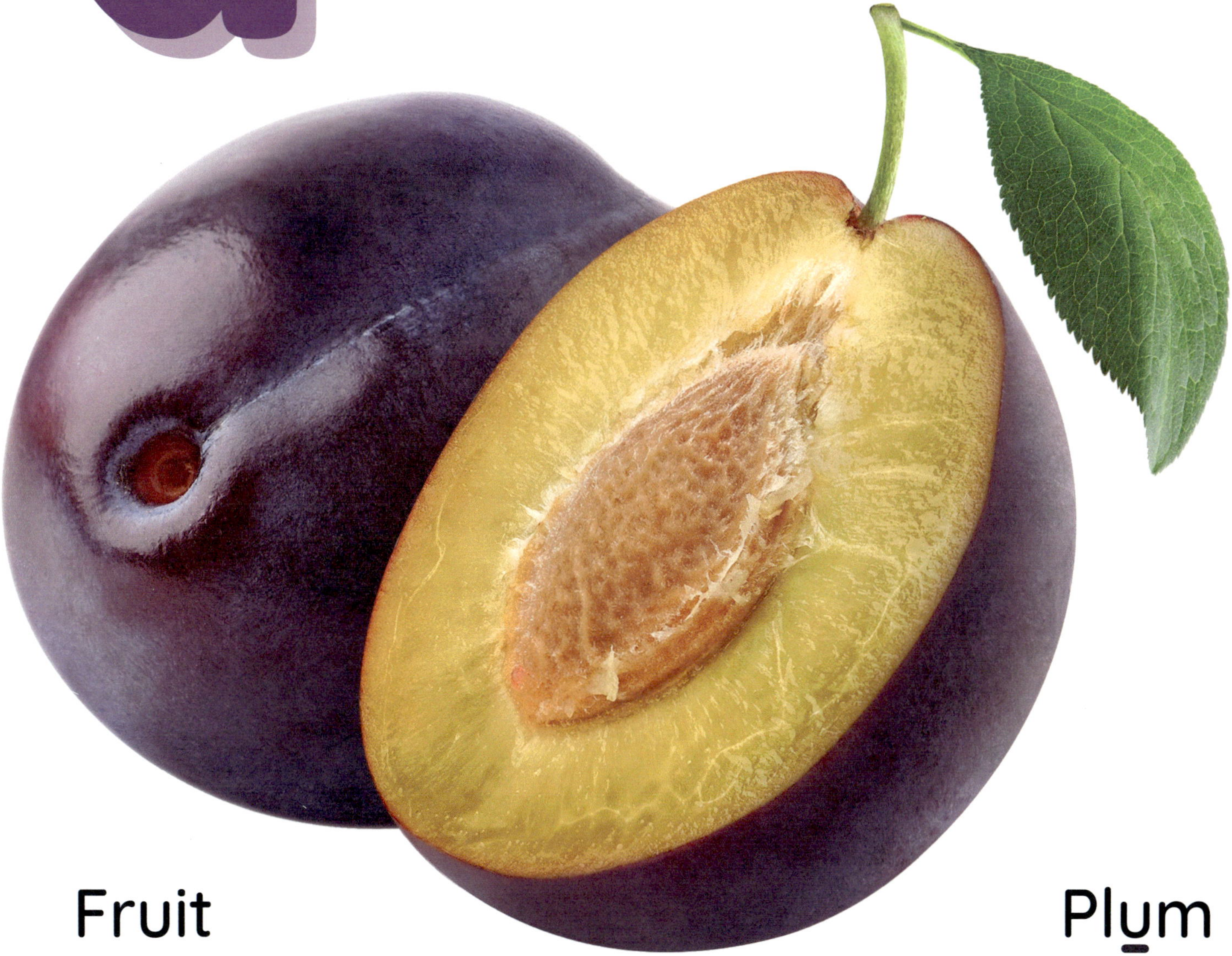

Fruit

Plum

V

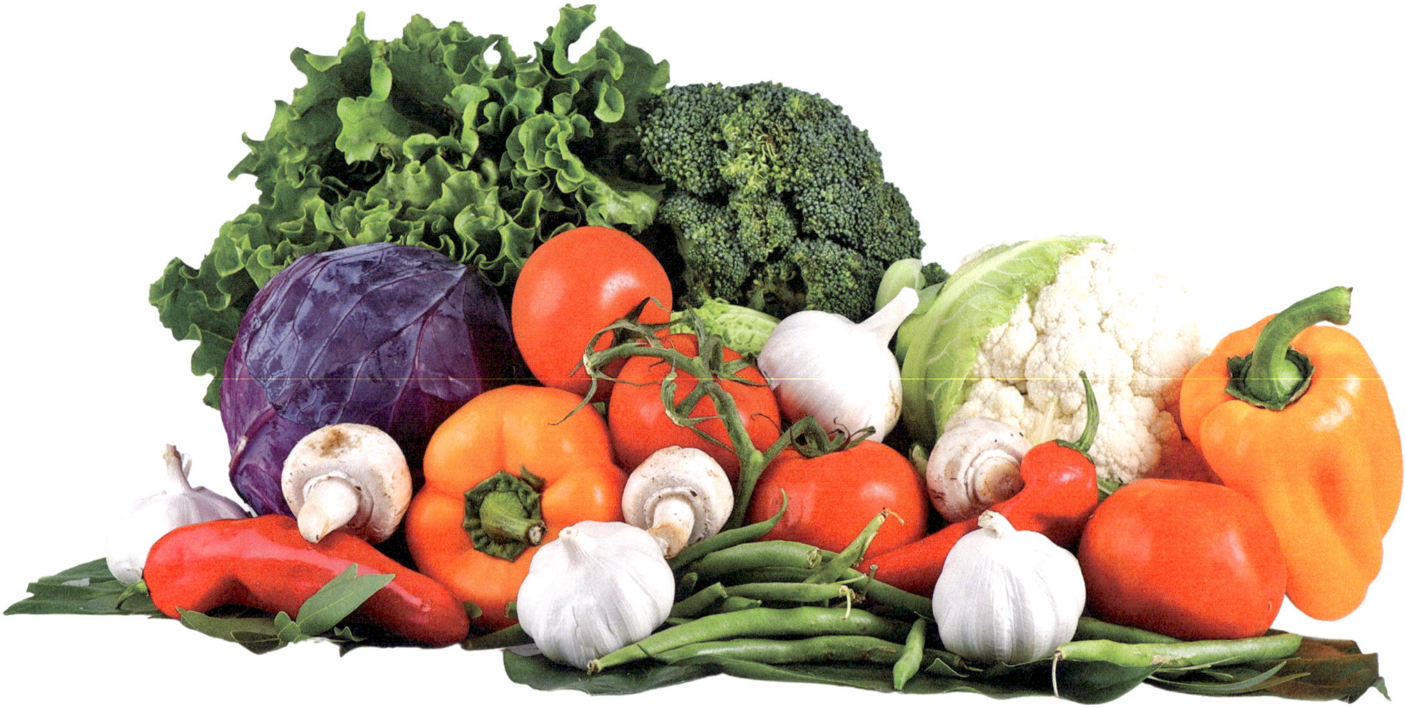

Vegetables

Vegetable

V

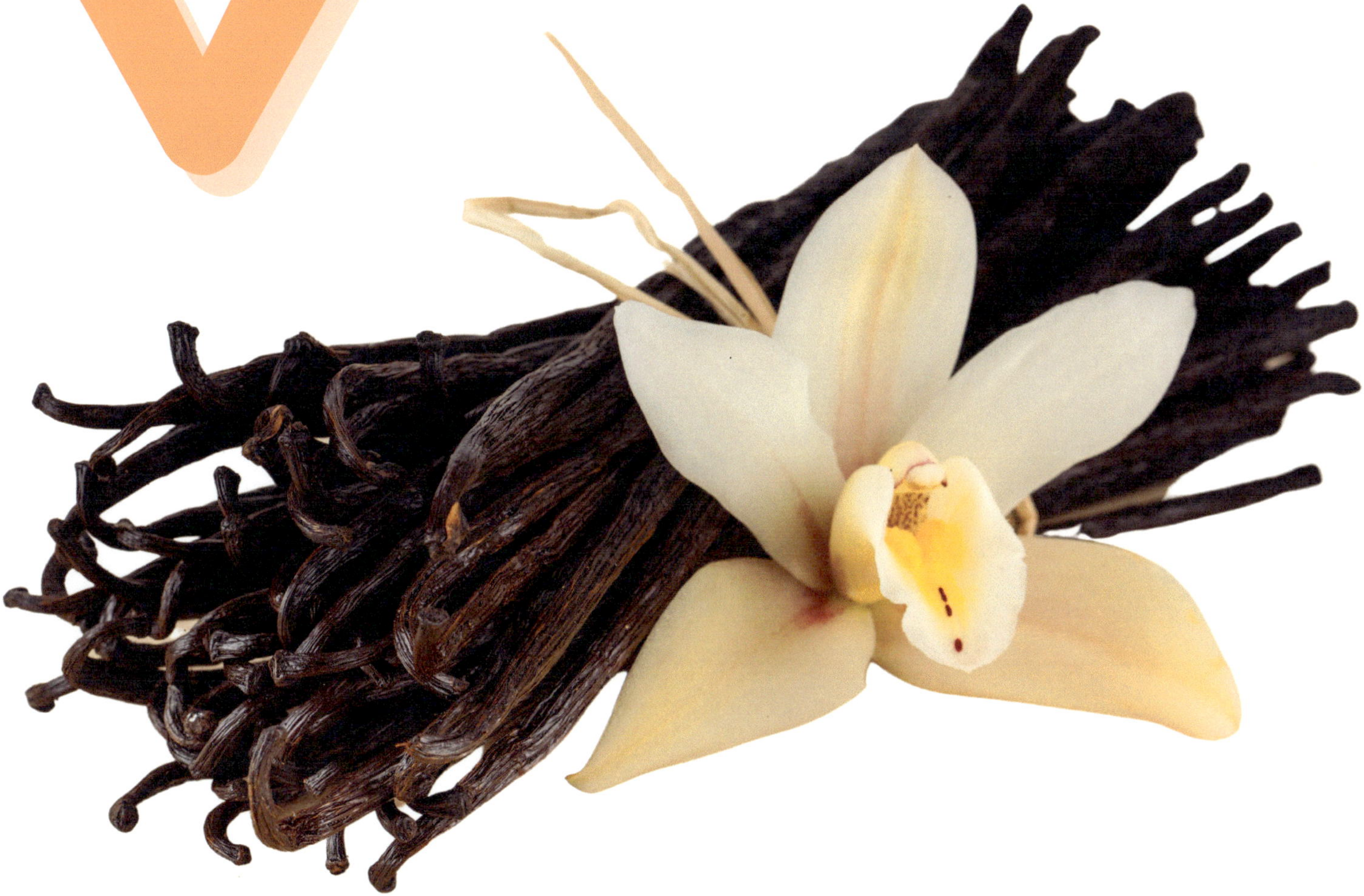

Fruit

Vanilla Bean

W

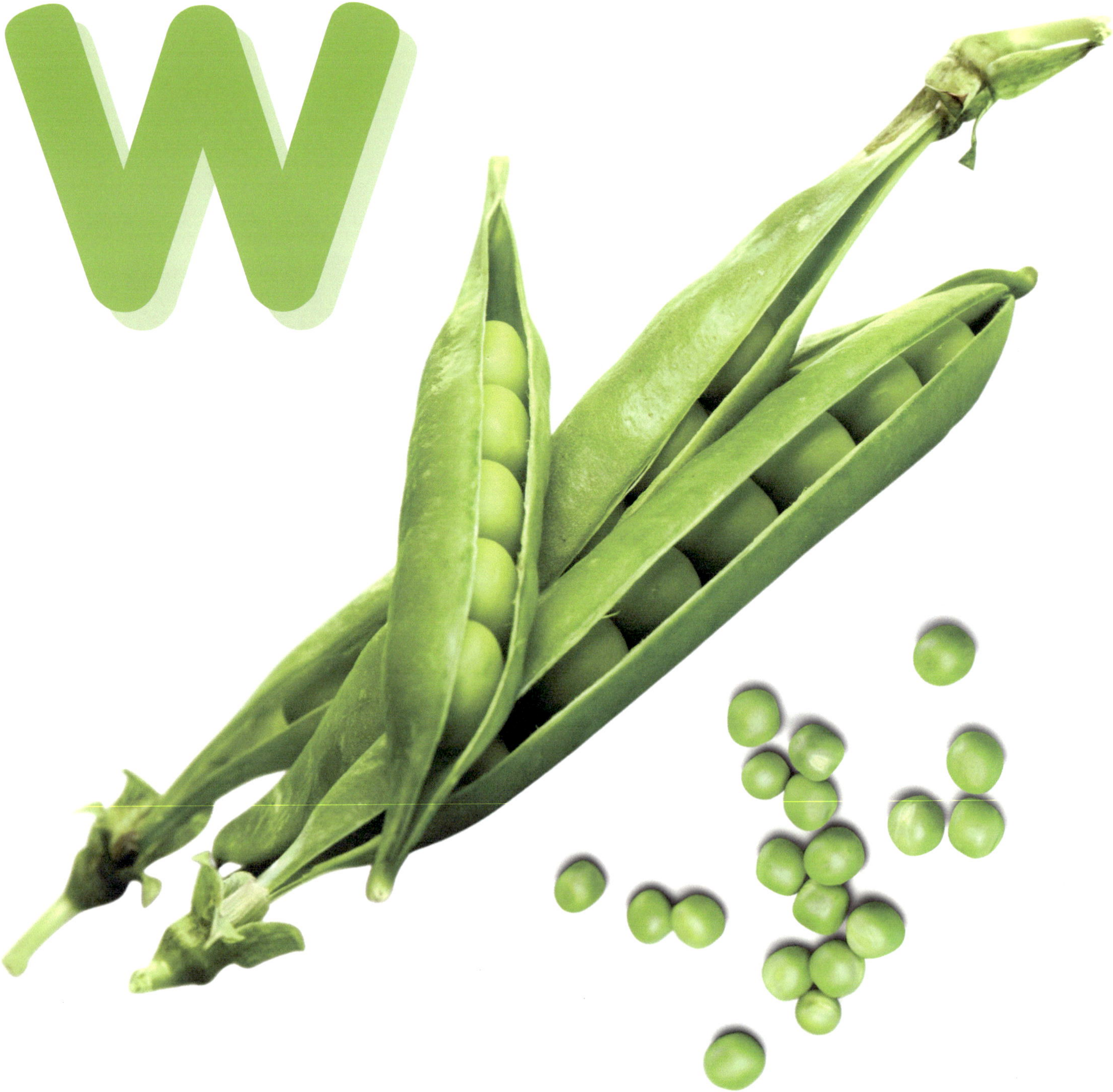

Snow Peas

Vegetable

W

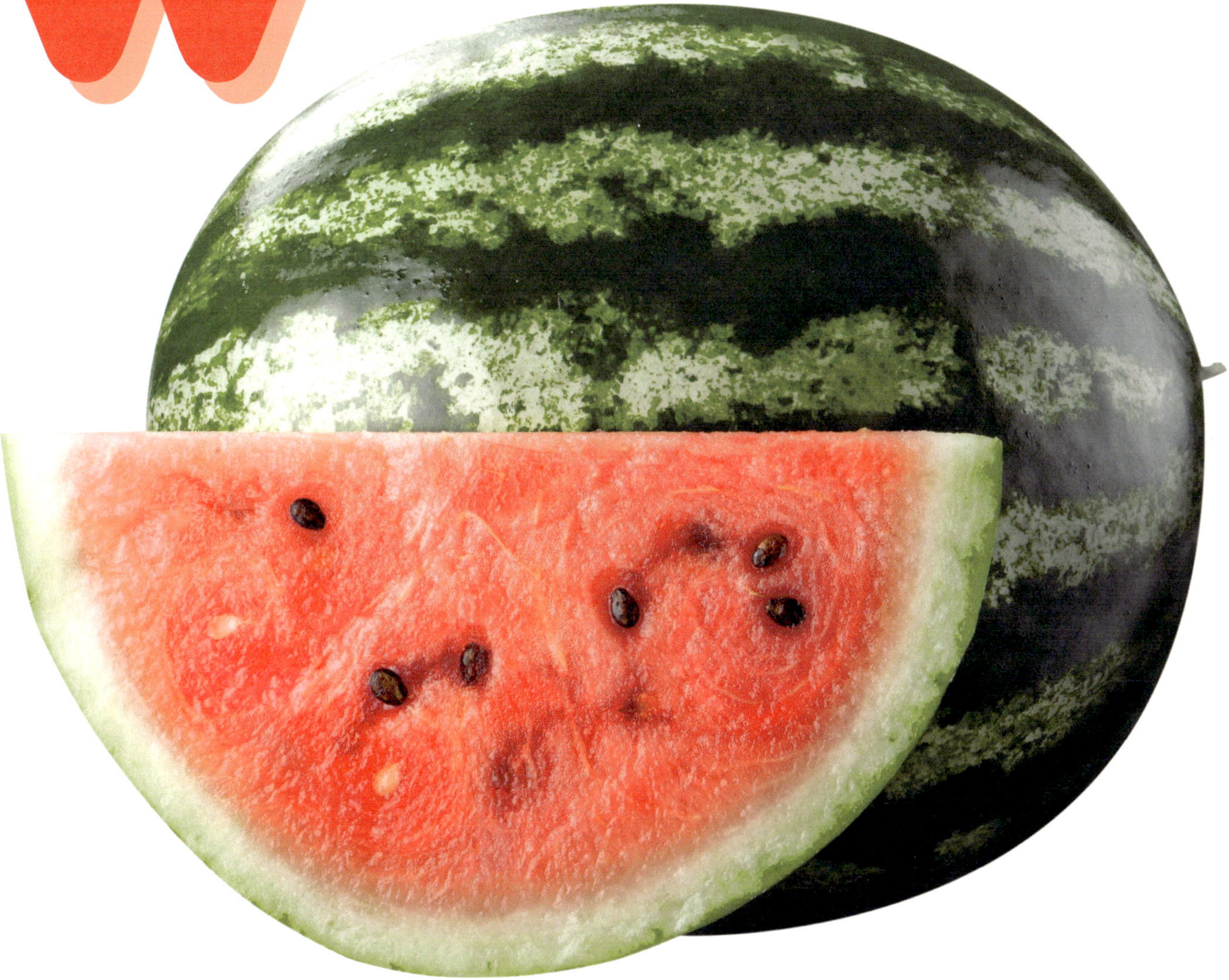

Fruit

Watermelon

X

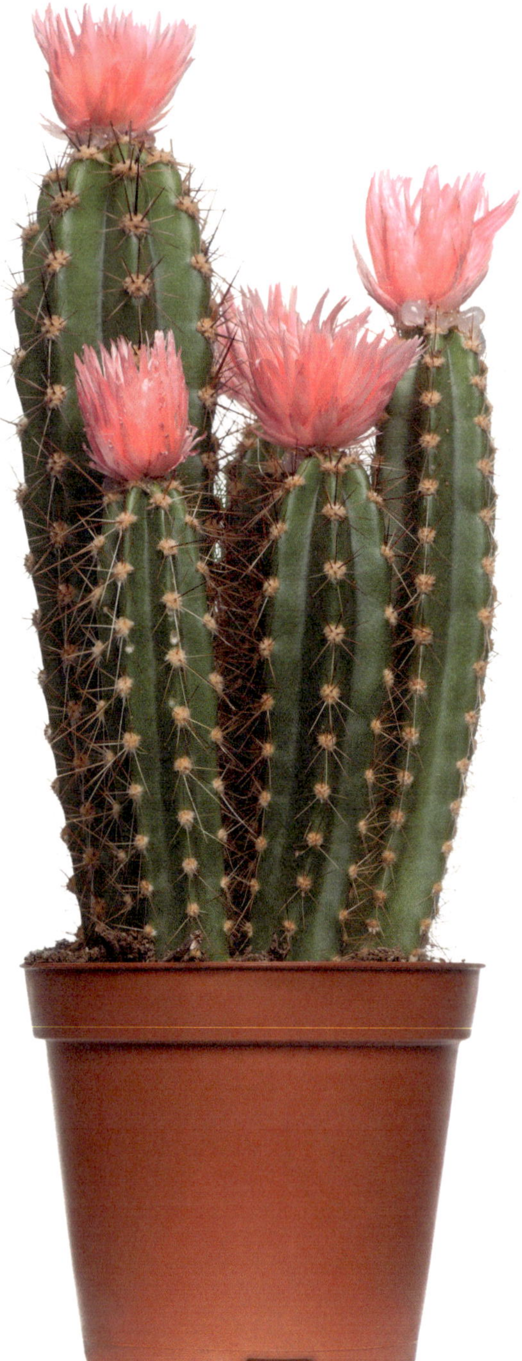

Mexican Cactus

Vegetable

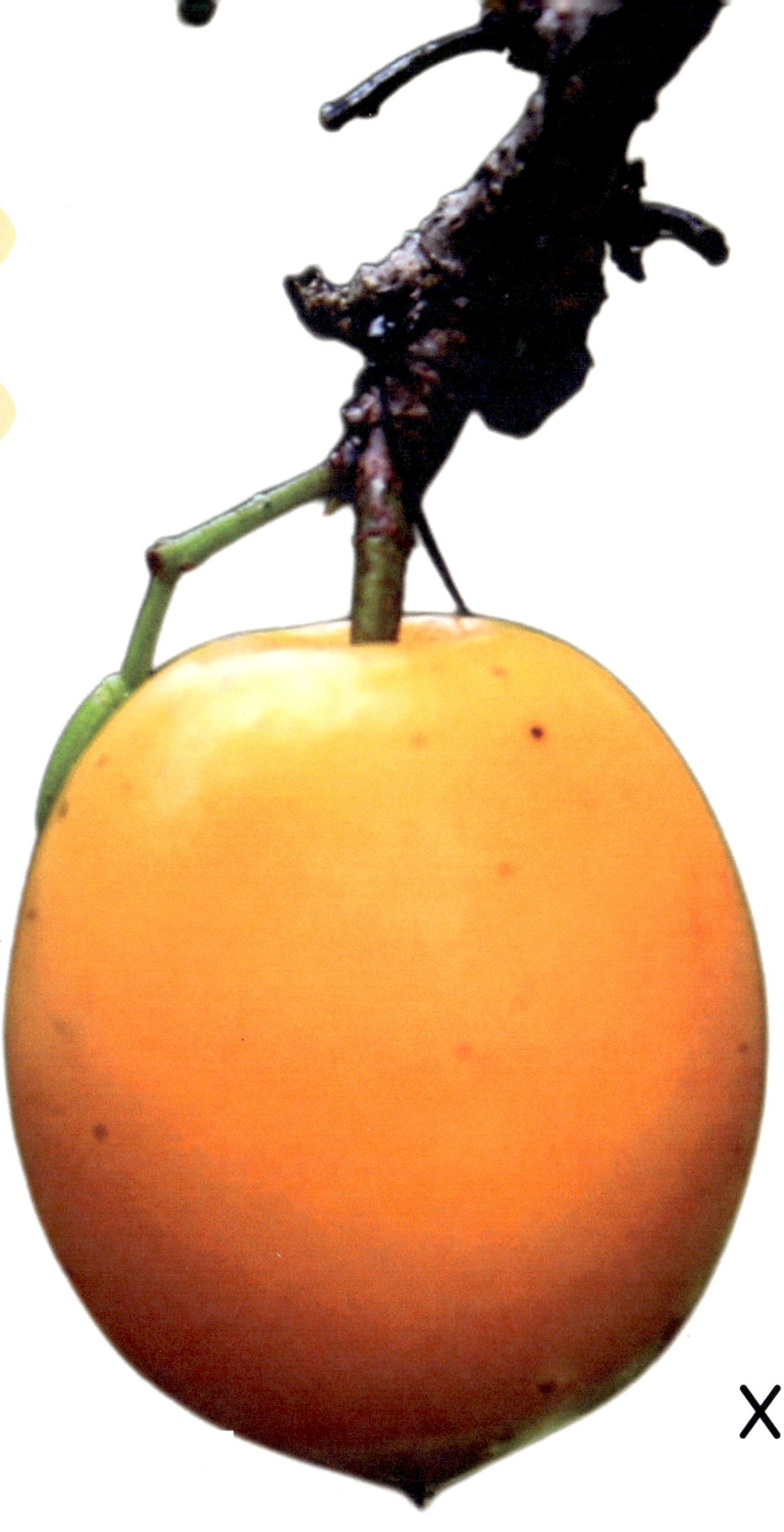

Fruit

Ximenia

Y

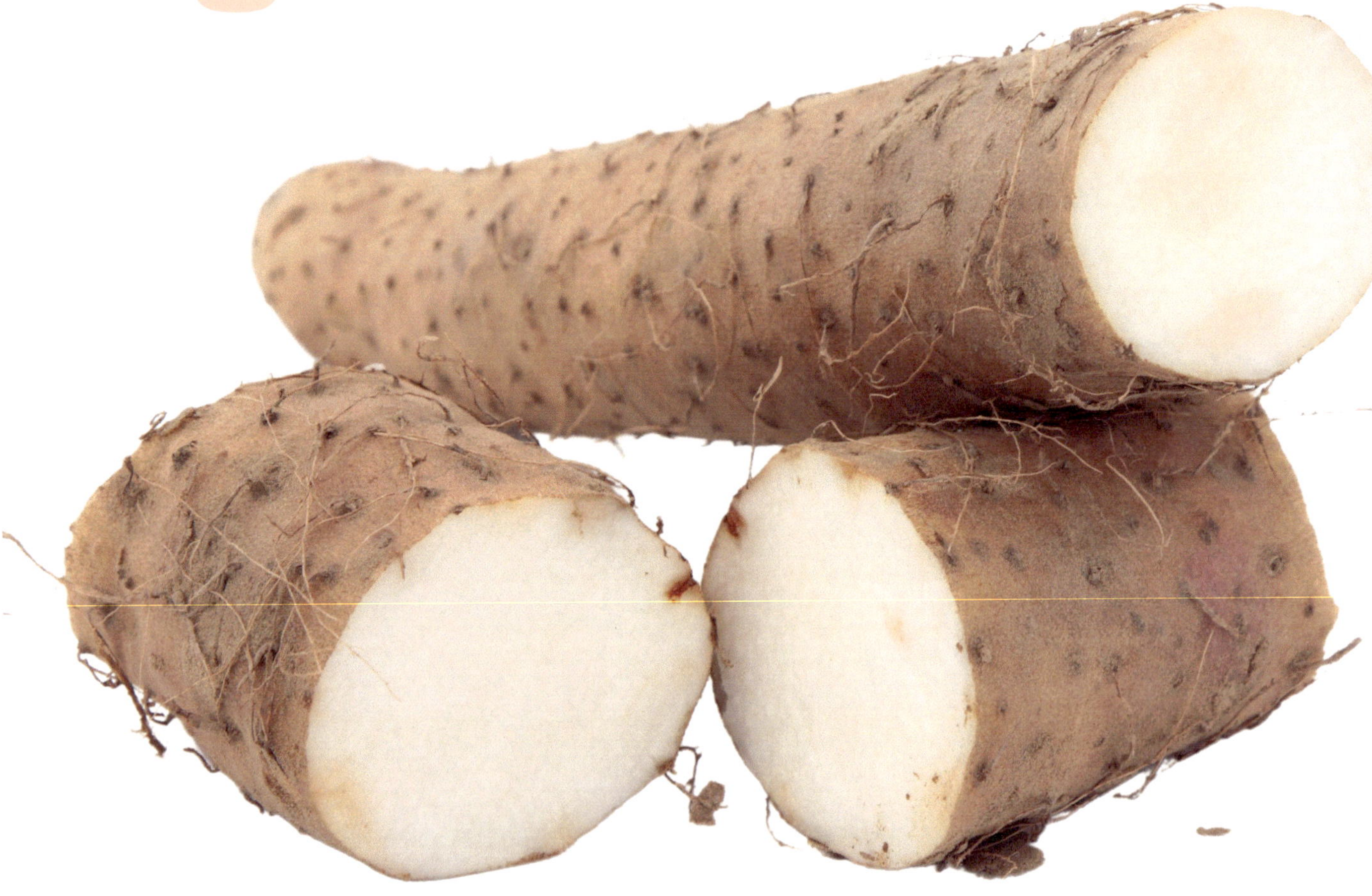

Yams

Vegetable

Y

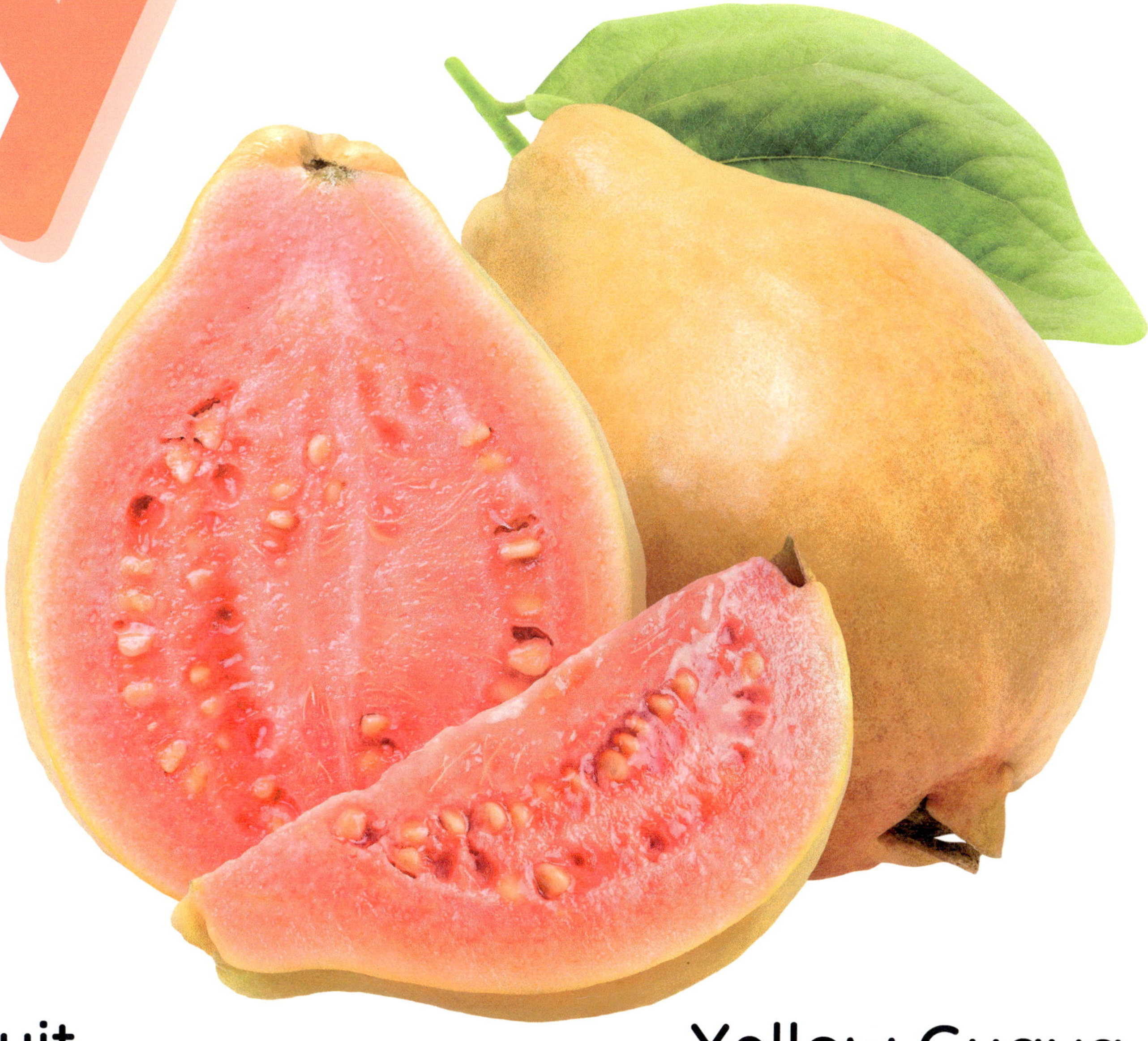

Fruit

Yellow Guava

Z

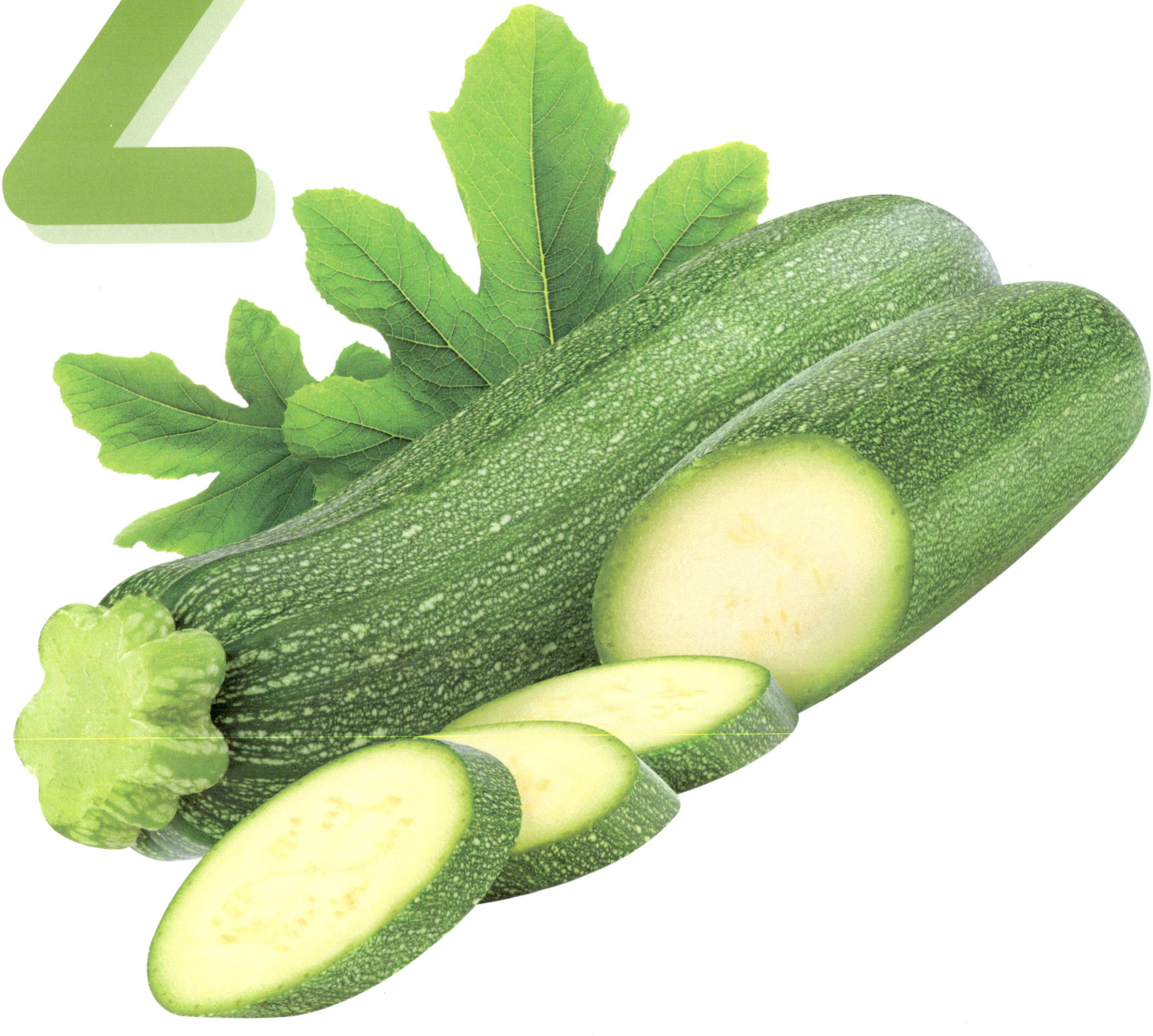

Zucchini

Vegetable

Z

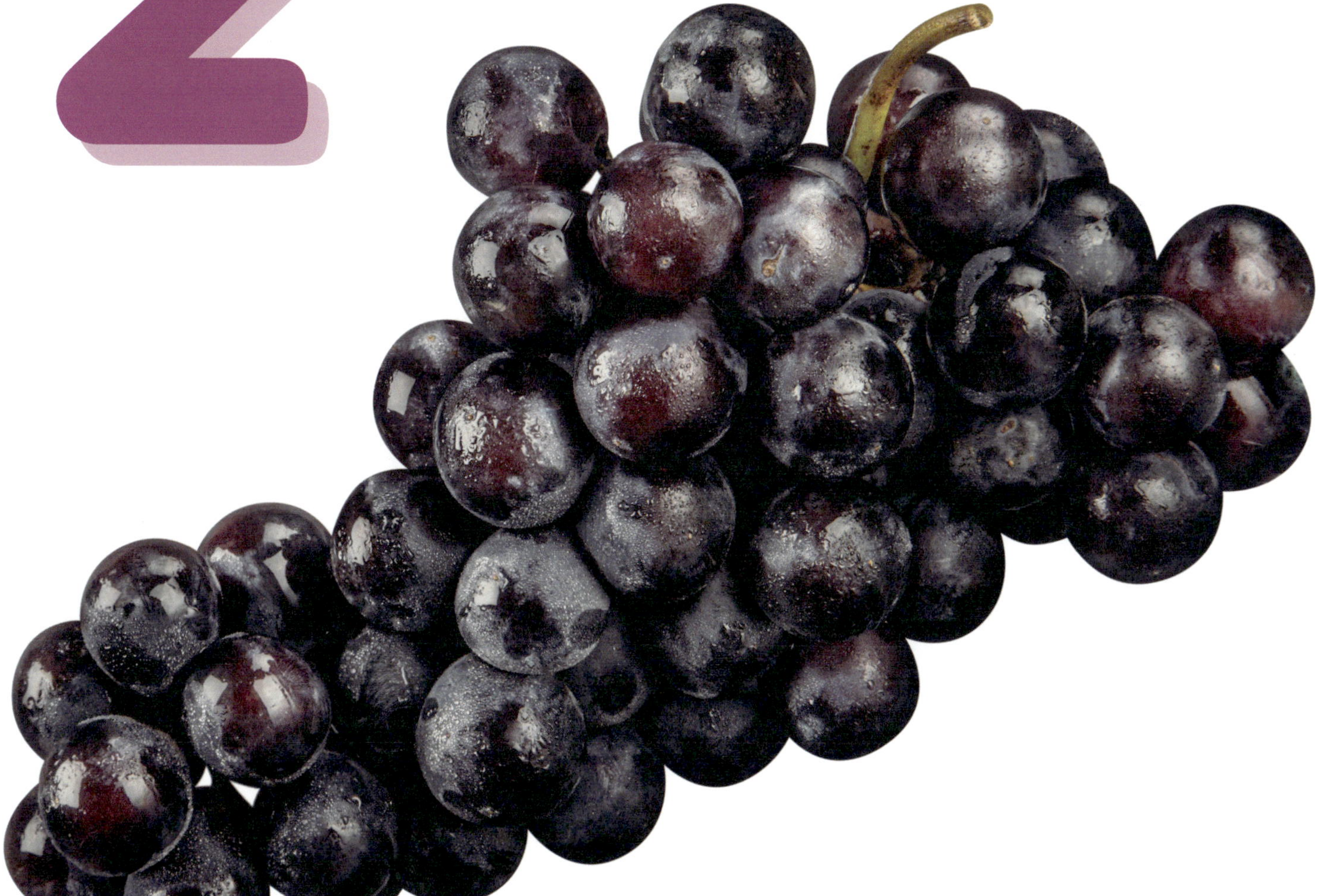

Fruit

Zinfandel Grapes

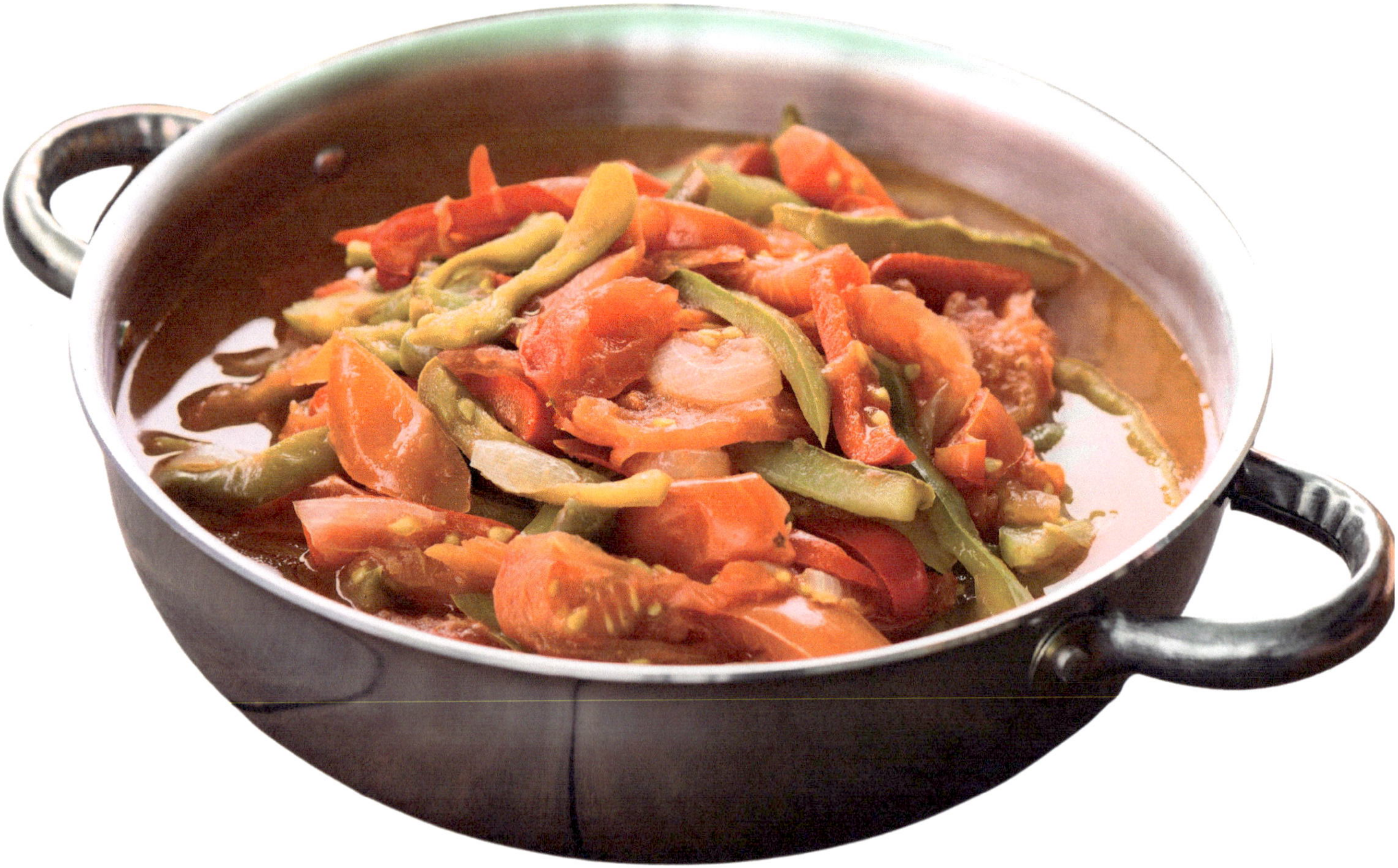

Veggie Stew

Vegetable

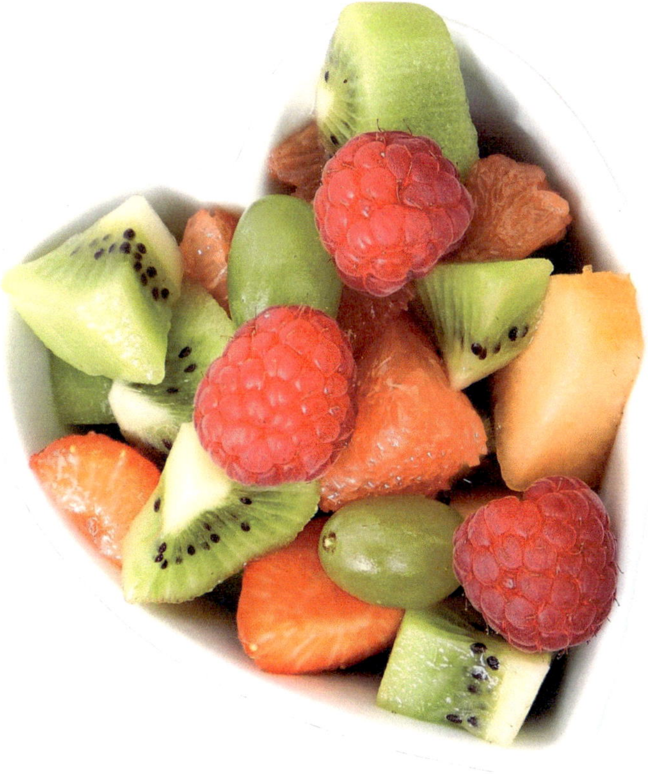

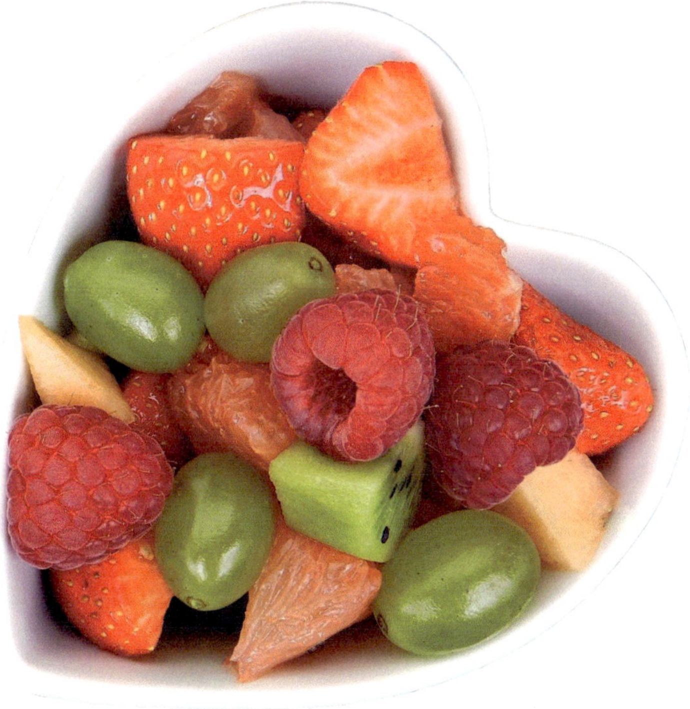

Fruit

Fruit Salad

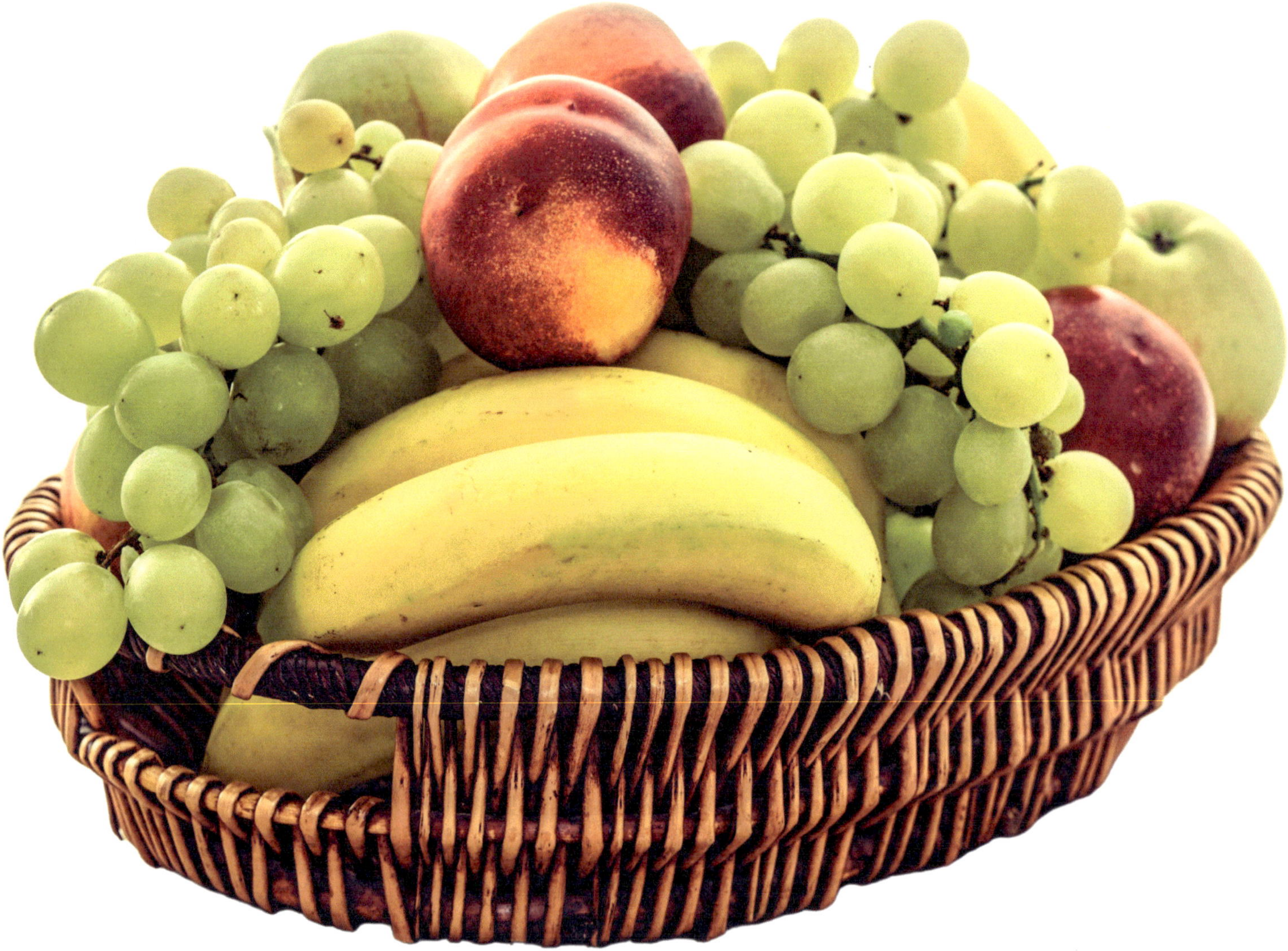

Fruit

Fruit Basket

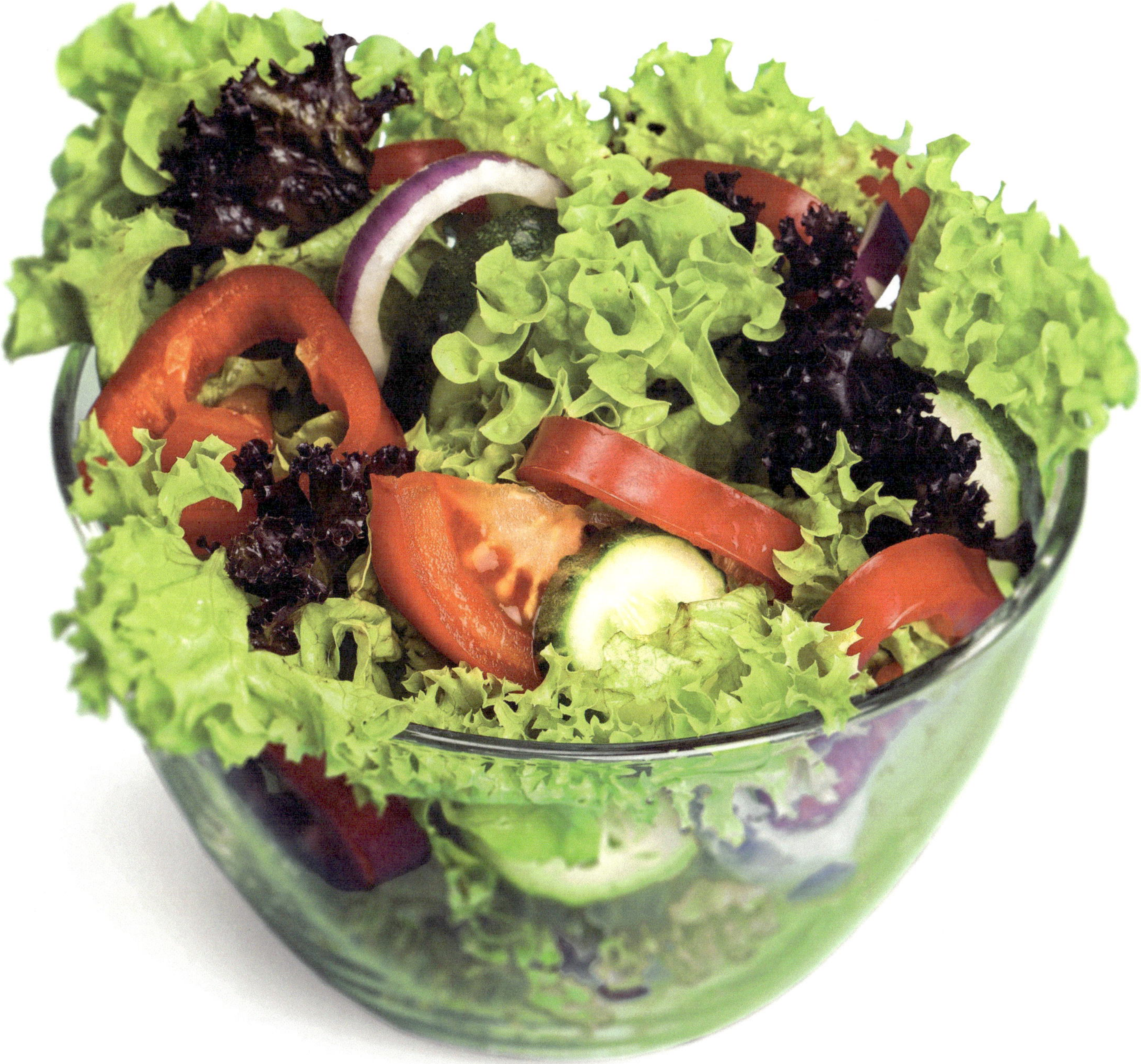

Salad Bowl

Vegetable

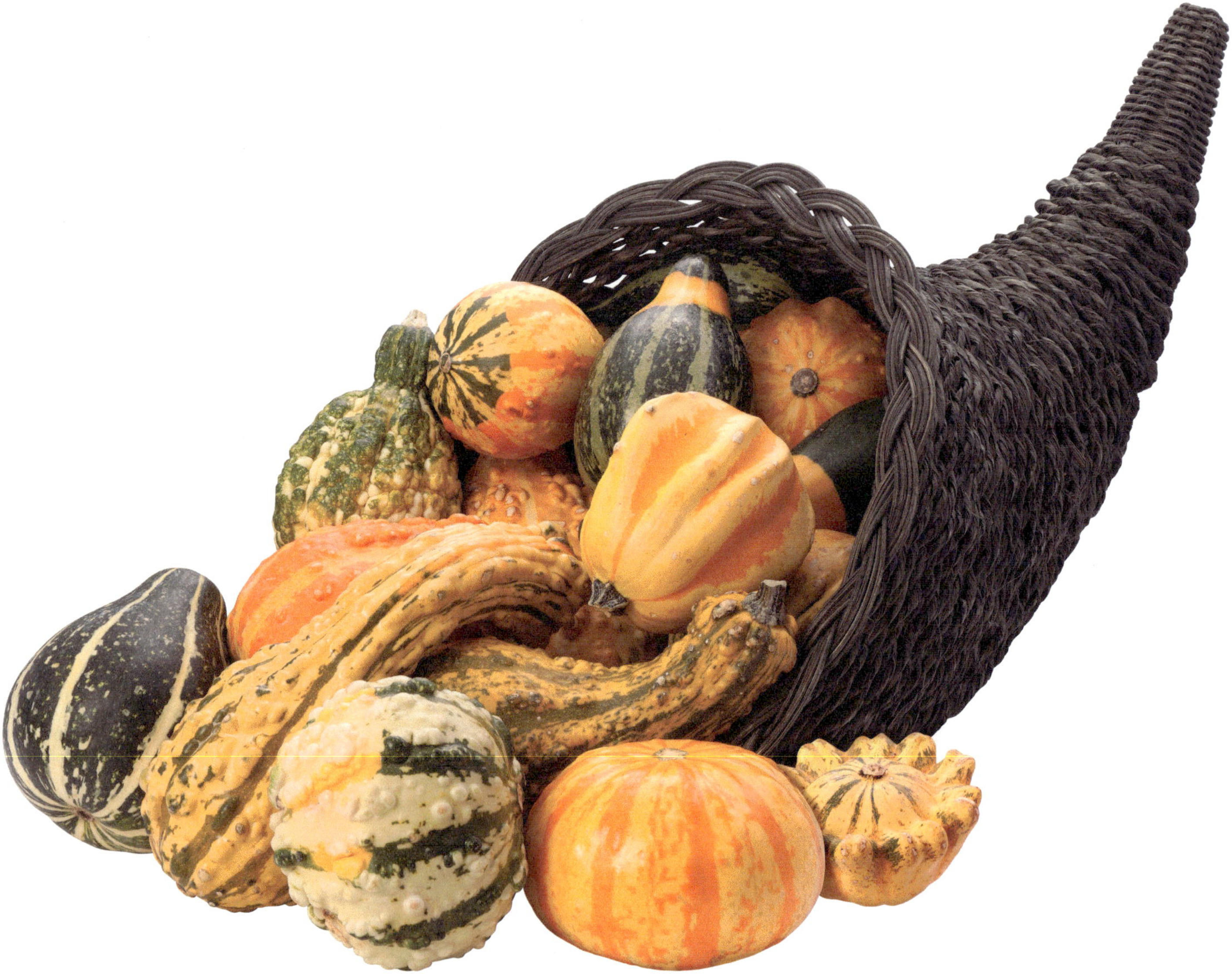

Cornicopia

Vegetable

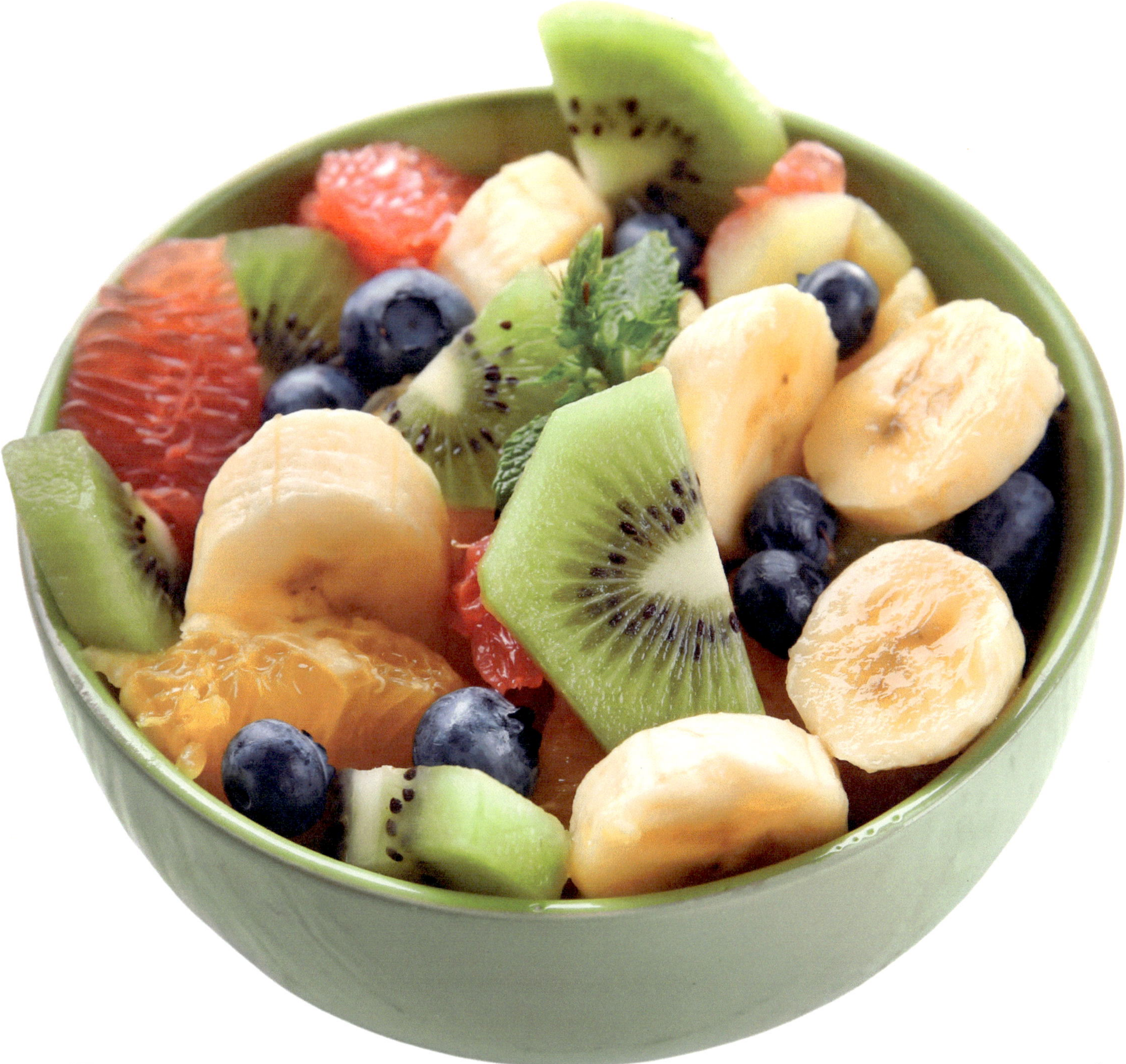

Fruit

Fruit Bowl

DRAW YOUR FAVORITE VEGGIE

DRAW YOUR FAVORITE FRUIT

THANK YOU

to all of our parents, kids, and adults who take the time to

REVIEW our books on Amazon.

Reviews really help us to better serve you.

Feel free to visit our website

www.WARMBLUSH.com

to view some of our other books

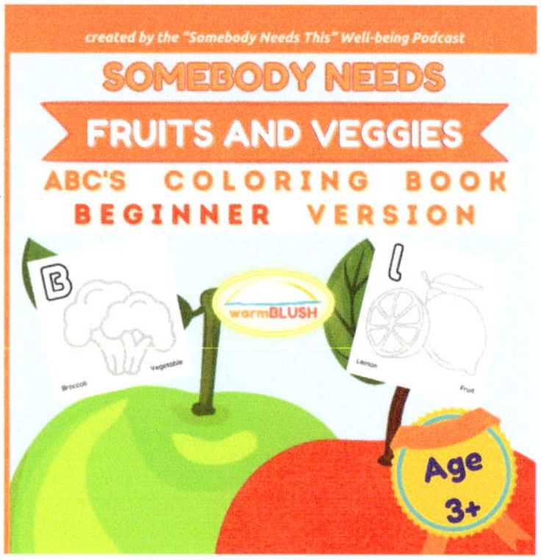

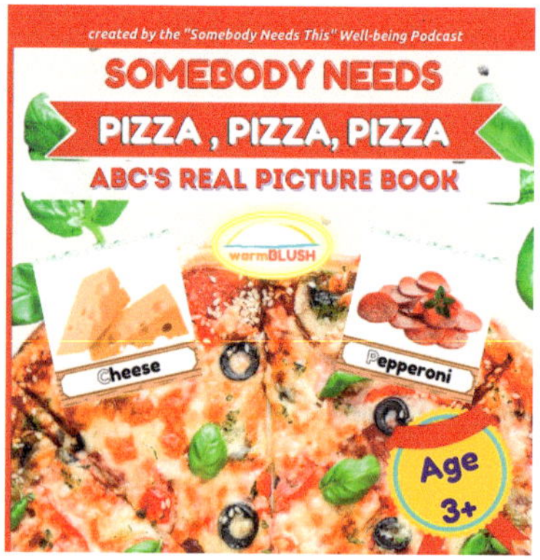

Made in the USA
Las Vegas, NV
08 November 2026

57691395R00040